The Complete
Pregnancy
Guide

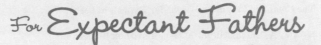

For Expectant Fathers

W9-BZQ-027

Everything a Dad Needs to Know About Pregnancy and Fatherhood

By Alex Lluch, Author of Over 4 Million Books Sold
& Dr. Benito Villanueva, M.D., Obstetrics and Gynecology

The Complete Pregnancy Guide for Expectant Fathers

By Alex A. Lluch, Author of Over 4 Million Books Sold
& Dr. Benito Villanueva, M.D., Obstetrics and Gynecology

Published by WS Publishing Group
San Diego, California
Copyright © 2012 by WS Publishing Group

All rights reserved under International and Pan-American Copyright conventions. No part of this book may be reproduced or transmitted in any form or by any means, electronic or mechanical, including photocopy, recording or by any information storage and retrieval system, without permission in writing from the publisher.

DISCLAIMER: The content in this book is provided for general informational purposes only and is not meant to substitute the advice provided by a medical professional. This information is not intended to diagnose or treat medical problems or substitute for appropriate medical care. Consult your physician before making any changes in your diet or exercise during pregnancy. If you or your partner are under the care of a physician and/or take medications for diabetes, heart disease, hypertension, or any other condition, consult your healthcare provider prior to initiation of any suggestions in this guide. If you have or suspect that you have a medical problem, promptly contact your healthcare provider. Never disregard professional medical advice or delay in seeking it because of something you have read in this book.

WS Publishing Group makes no claims whatsoever regarding the interpretation or utilization of any information contained herein and/or recorded by the user of this book. If you utilize any information provided in this book, you do so at your own risk and you specifically waive any right to make any claim against the author and publisher, its officers, directors, employees or representatives as the result of the use of such information.

For Inquiries:
Visit www.WSPublishingGroup.com
E-mail info@WSPublishingGroup.com

ISBN: 978-1-936061-30-3

Printed in China

. . . . Table of Contents

Table of Contents. . . . . 🦆

Table of Contents

DEDICATED TO FATHERS-TO-BE EVERYWHERE.
MAY THESE MONTHS BE
THE MOST EXCITING OF YOUR LIFE!

Introduction

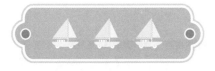

Congratulations!

IN A SPEECH GIVEN ON FATHER'S DAY 2008, Barack Obama, then the Democratic presidential nominee, said, "Of all the rocks upon which we build our lives, we are reminded today that family is the most important. And we are called to recognize and honor how critical every father is to that foundation. They are teachers and coaches. They are mentors and role models. They are examples of success and the men who constantly push us toward it." As a man who made his way to impressive heights despite growing up with an absentee father, he said he desired but one thing: "that if I could be anything in life, I would be a good father to my girls; that if I could give them anything, I would give them that rock—that foundation—on which to build their lives. And that would be the greatest gift I could offer." Obama's words are a resounding call to action for every man who has just learned he is going to be a father.

In years past, the role of a father was deemed secondary, even irrelevant, to motherhood, and certainly during pregnancy. But fathers-to-be now live in a world where it has been scientifically proven that fatherhood is just as important to a child's development as motherhood. It has taken much time and many revelations by researchers to learn this lesson, but, as a new dad, you will benefit from the societal evolution of parenting. The support, encouragement, and love you give your partner during this time is critical to your baby's development in utero. Your bonding as parents-to-be, the sound of your voice, and the effort and energy you bring to your household all have profound effects upon your baby's development.

THE REWARDS OF FATHERHOOD

Fatherhood is the most rewarding job you will have in your lifetime. Not only do you get to shape and nurture a tiny person from infancy to adulthood, but you become a better, healthier man in the process.

Upon hearing the news that your partner is pregnant, your eyes are suddenly opened wide to all of the ways in which life must change in order to live up to your expectations of fatherhood. Responding to this realization is often how an expectant father spends the majority of his partner's pregnancy, which has the added bonus of lasting health benefits. Common ways this plays out include using this time to quit smoking, cut down on alcohol consumption, give up using illegal drugs, start or continue an exercise plan, eat a healthy diet, visit the doctor for a physical, get more sleep, and reduce your stress levels.

Making these changes during pregnancy improves your immediate physical health. But in the longer term it also gives you the energy and stamina to keep up with your child over the years and be actively involved throughout your child's life. Moreover, making healthier choices during pregnancy shows solidarity with your partner, who is physically forced to make significant lifestyle changes. This results in a deeply intimate connection with your partner that will carry over for the rest of your lives together. As Antoine de Saint-Expurey, author of The Little Prince, wisely observed, "Love does not consist of gazing at each other, but in looking together in the same direction." This is, perhaps, the greatest advertisement of all for the close participation of the expectant father in his partner's pregnancy.

THE EXCITEMENT OF PREGNANCY FOR FATHERS-TO-BE

Finding out your partner is pregnant is one of the single most exciting moments in your life. If you have been battling infertility, the positive sign on the pregnancy test wand will be welcome relief from fertility treatments, having to constantly assure your partner that everything will work out, and gives you and your partner a break from "functional" sex—that is, sex for the sole purpose of conceiving.

On the other hand, if you and your partner became pregnant soon after making the decision to "go for it," you are probably relieved that it worked out so quickly. Finally, if you were not expecting to become a father this soon, there is a part of you that is amazed, impressed, and excited.

This excitement is usually followed swiftly by unmitigated fear for men. Usually this fear mounts by quickly calculating all the ways in which your life is about to change. And change it will—having a baby affects everything, from your relationship with your partner, to your career, to your friendships, and possibly even your world outlook and politics. This is because issues that did not concern you before suddenly matter more than anything else. Examples are the condition of the schools in your area, affordable daycare, breast-feeding in public, and toy safety standards. Your shifting concerns, interests, and responsibilities can cause your relationships to change with those in your community who do not have children. This can be a difficult transition, but ultimately, your friends and

Introduction . . . .

family will adjust along with you and love your child almost as much as you do. And of course, all of these adjustments are worth it, as there is possibly nothing as grand in this world as being a parent.

Having a baby turns your family of two into a family of three or more. The addition of people to your family is challenging to manage for both fathers, mothers, and older children. However, with some careful time management skills, good communication, and a commitment to retain your identity as a couple, you will not only get through this transition, but will forge deeper connections than those that existed before. After all, there are many decisions that you must make together as your pregnancy progresses and your baby's arrival draws near.

Many men are unable to anticipate how expecting a child will highlight other absences in their lives, such as the loss of a partner, sibling, parent, or previous pregnancies. It is perfectly normal to mourn these losses as if they were fresh when filled with all of this new potential. It is to be expected that you would want to share this news and the life of your child with those who have passed away and are still dear to you. Learning that you are expecting a child will likely heighten your respect—now more than ever—for the cycle of life and death and help you to appreciate the wonder and joy that is coming in just 10 months.

A BRIEF EXPLANATION OF MOM'S ESTIMATED DUE DATE

As you get a handle on your thoughts about becoming a father, you are probably wondering when it will all begin. Your partner's estimated due date (EDD) will be calculated by her doctor according to when the first day of her last menstrual period (LMP) was. According to LMP calculations, your partner's estimated due date (EDD) is 40 weeks from the first day of her last period, or 280 days.

However, your partner is not actually pregnant for all of that time. She is not officially pregnant until a fertilized egg implants into her uterus. Therefore, actual gestation—the time between conception and birth—lasts 38 weeks, or 266 days. Either way, mom's estimated due date will be the same. For example, if your partner's period started on November 1, her EDD will be August 8.

In this book, coverage of the changes happening to mom's body and of baby's development is measured in lunar months. Each lunar month consists of 28 days broken down into 4 weeks, with 7 days each. This means your partner will be pregnant for 10 lunar months, but this is only an estimate for when baby will be born. You can use the EDD for planning purposes, but don't get married to it. Only 5 percent of babies are actually born on their EDD. More common are babies who are born in the 3 weeks before and 2 weeks after mom's due date.

"If you want one year of prosperity, grow grain. If you want ten years of prosperity, grow trees. If you want one hundred years of prosperity, grow babies."
~ Chinese Proverb

Notes . . . .

What to Expect

A CLASSIC QUOTE FROM WINNIE THE POOH advises, "Before beginning a Hunt, it is wise to ask someone what you are looking for before you begin looking for it." This is a wise sentiment for any man to keep in mind as he prepares for fatherhood. Indeed, before you tackle all of the life changes and issues encompassed by fatherhood, you first must understand what they are. The way to do that is to learn all you can about what to expect during pregnancy. Reading this step-by-step guide will help you, as will talking with other dads, and participating in pregnancy 100 percent of the time. Only then will you begin to understand the Great Hunt for successful parenting.

WHAT TO EXPECT FROM FATHERHOOD

Fatherhood is a journey that continues throughout your child's life, and indeed, throughout your own. Therefore, you should expect to constantly adjust your lifestyle to accommodate the various stages your family finds itself in. This book illuminates both the obvious and hidden issues that will require your attention before conception, during pregnancy, and into the first six weeks after your son or daughter is born.

What to Expect . . . .

DIFFERENT KINDS OF DADS

The journey through fatherhood is an individual one. Therefore, no two men react to it in the same way. There are men who take to the idea immediately, and those who require time to adjust. If you are among the latter—and most common—group of men, you will probably feel inadequately prepared to be a dad at first. But doubting your readiness and ability to be a father is normal. It is a good idea to use pregnancy as a time to ease into the idea. Allow the type of father you are reveal itself to you over time. Indeed, the worst thing you can do is to try to rush into becoming the kind of dad you think should be, instead of being the one that you are.

What does this mean in practice? It means that instead of forcing yourself to be the "can't wait for baby" guy, let yourself hang out in the "I'm not ready for fatherhood" zone for awhile. If it takes you longer to settle in your new reality than you (or your partner) expected, do not take this as a sign that you are not ready to be a parent. Rather, be patient and understand that your feelings about fatherhood will constantly evolve throughout your partner's pregnancy. For example, it is possible that you will start out being incredibly excited and supportive—only to see these feelings taper off in the second trimester when mom seems to need you less. Or, you may begin pregnancy nervous and panicky, only to find that in just a few months you feel calm and in control. Be reassured that no matter what emotions you had during the course of pregnancy, you will feel just one overriding emotion the day your child is born: sheer joy.

Until then, though, it is likely that you may be most affected by fear—fear of miscarriage, fear of labor and childbirth, fear of losing your partner, fear of being a family instead of a couple, fear of the added financial burdens—the list is nearly endless. It is helpful, in this case, to identify what your concerns are, deal with them, and move on.

For example, men who have poor relationships with their fathers are often terrified of repeating the same mistakes with their own child. Get over this fear by acknowledging the disappointments of this relationship. Then spend some time thinking about the ways in which that relationship, though hurtful, has taught you about the kind of father you want to be. Make the decision to not let this relationship be the only one that shapes your parenting style. Instead, look to other family members and friends whom you respect for guidance. Recognizing other, more positive male role models you have had in your life will keep your fears and doubts in check.

Limiting the degree to which you allow fear to lord over your other pregnancy-related emotions is necessary to your entire family's well-being. Consider how it feels to be afraid—your muscles are constantly tensed, your sleep poorly, you suffer from headaches, and your appetite is erratic. None of these symptoms help your ability to grow into your new role as a dad. Besides, your disposition will affect how your partner feels and may cause unnecessary tension between the two of you. It is therefore in your family's best interest to experience, explore, and then allow fear to exit your consciousness within a reasonable amount of time. This makes room for other feelings to have a turn at the surface, such as joy and anticipation.

Interestingly, even once anxiety is under control, many dads-to-be experience guarded excitement until the end of the first trimester, and then again during the third. If this sounds like you, it is likely that you are thrilled about having a baby but terrified of miscarriage or the loss of baby and/or your partner during delivery. Thus, just as your nerves give way to fantasies of throwing a baseball with your son, the crushing anxiety that something will happen to prevent this from becoming a reality crashes in. Something to keep in mind is that your partner feels exactly the same way. Furthermore, just having these thoughts and feelings means you have already begun your journey as a father! Indeed, you will experience both excitement and anxiety each time your child reaches a milestone—when they are born, on their first day of school, when they go to their first dance, the day they learn to drive, and when you send them off to college. So, it makes perfect sense to find yourself experiencing those same feelings at the very beginning of your child's life.

FINANCES

Though you should be fiscally responsible and have a general financial plan in place, try not to let money rule your thoughts of fatherhood. While it is true that having a child is an expensive experience, it is also a priceless one. As Ralph Waldo Emerson once wrote, "Can anybody remember when the times were not hard and money not scarce?" Many couples are so worried about the expense of parenthood that they wait until they have "enough" money to try and have a baby. But what is enough? If you wait until you are financially prepared to have a baby, it is quite possible you will never get to it. That said, there are costs that you can plan for both before and after your baby is born. Learning what these are can help you approach fatherhood with your heart rather than your wallet.

First get acquainted with the medical costs of pregnancy, since they are your immediate concern. The most consistent medical costs during pregnancy are the prenatal visits. On average, normal pregnancies require that moms see their OB-GYN once a month at first and then every one or two weeks until delivery. Depending on your partner's health and the type of insurance you have, pregnancy costs can range from minimal to very expensive.

If you have an HMO with a co-pay, these visits are not expected to break your bank. However, some co-insurance plans require up to 30 percent of the cost of each appointment and diagnostic test to be paid by the patient. Also, if your partner suffers from secondary conditions that require medication, bed rest, additional doctor's visits, or early hospitalization, your medical bills can become mountainous. Therefore, one of your first jobs as a dad is to contact your insurance company to find out exactly what is covered and what your financial responsibilities are. (When you call, ask for the name of the person you speak with, write it down, and have it handy in case discrepancies arise later on.) Knowing what you are in for will take the "shock and awe" out of opening your medical bills.

Your second job is to find out what portion of the hospital stay you are responsible for when your partner is ready to deliver. In general, many plans require a "flat fee" or co-pay of $250 to $500 upon hospital admittance. Considering that the average cost of having a baby in the United States is more than $8,000, if you have to pay $250—or even $1,000—consider yourself lucky. This fee usually covers medications, hospital charges, and emergency medical interventions associated with the birth of your child.

If you are still not satisfied after speaking to your insurance representative, get online. Most insurance companies have their policies online and organized by topic. Click on anything that says "pregnancy," print it out, and read it. If you still have questions, ask them well before your partner is admitted to the hospital. Also, talk to your doctor about pre-registering at the hospital to give the administration time to process your insurance in case there are any blips in your plan.

If you are one of the thousands of uninsured Americans who are facing pregnancy, do not panic. There are several state-run programs that offer financial assistance for prenatal care, labor, and delivery. Your doctor will be able to give you suggestions for where to find such programs, as will health organizations like Planned Parenthood.

While you are dealing with insurance issues, take the time to increase your life insurance plan or to put one in place. Obtaining life insurance for yourself and your partner is one of the first ways in which you assert your responsibility as a parent—in other words, it's an active way of acknowledging that your life is no longer just about you. While most young people consider insurance to be a morbid, even irrelevant topic, it is important to make sure your child has something in place should the worst happen.

Most first-time parents purchase "term life insurance." It is the least expensive plan that insures you for a fixed amount at a set premium. As your income increases or your family grows you can increase the amount you are insured by paying a higher premium. If you already had life insurance, now is a good opportunity to update any information that has changed. You should also reevaluate the beneficiaries specified in your will and choose guardians for your child in the event both you and your partner die before your child turns 18. These are by no means pleasant topics to deal with—but the idea of your child having to make do without such protections in place is worse.

Finally, in addition to medical and insurance costs, you should be prepared to make several big purchases before you bring your baby home. For starters, your partner will eventually need maternity clothes. It is hard to say when—it depends on how big she gets and how early she begins to show. A word of advice: never suggest to your partner "it looks like it's time" for maternity clothes. Instead, let her splurge now and then on something that makes her feel good about herself. Letting her determine what she wears and when she wears it will save you from many tearful arguments! In addition to new threads for mom, you will need a crib, car seat, stroller, some starter diapers, clothes for baby, and infant formula if your partner does not plan to breast-feed. The car seat is a must above all musts—the hospital will not let you take your baby home without one. These are just some of the costs you can expect to incur over the next year. It is a good idea to start a pregnancy savings account, or at the very least, cut back on a fancy dinner here and there to save up.

CHANGES IN YOUR RELATIONSHIP

There is, perhaps, no greater force of change for a relationship than pregnancy. You can ease the transition from duo to trio (or more) by going along with changes instead of trying to prevent them. As Charles Darwin once wrote, "It is not the strongest of the species that survives, nor the most intelligent, but the one most responsive to change." And change your family will. Since pregnancy forces your family to alter how it spends, eats, socializes, divides household duties, and manages its health, you will find that being flexible is the key to survival! Indeed, pregnancy—though a time of great hope and joy—is also riddled with bouts of intense stress that may affect the way you and your partner communicate and experience intimacy. It may even alter your identity as a couple.

One reason pregnancy puts stress on a relationship is because much of dad's time is spent trying to anticipate his partner's needs while simultaneously dealing with his own feelings about becoming a father. This can cause emotions to "bottleneck," or cram together like a train that has run off its track. This intense crash of emotion may affect how you communicate with your partner. In fact, for many couples it can feel like they are suddenly speaking completely different languages! This is due in part to people applying their usual methods of interaction to completely unfamiliar circumstances. Learning new ways to communicate with your pregnant partner, therefore, is necessary to surviving her sometimes volatile state.

For example, if you can avoid becoming defensive when she is inexplicably angry, you may end up laughing rather than fighting about whatever it was that made her mad. If you can learn to save your teasing for when she no longer feels unattractive and fat, you can avoid hurting her feelings and causing a damaging argument. However, if you insist on fighting when she is clearly agitated, or you tend to snap when she is weepy, you are in for a long and difficult pregnancy!

In addition to communication, many pregnant couples also experience shifts in intimacy. This is largely dictated by how your partner feels on a given day—or even in a particular moment— which can make you feel powerless and sidelined. Try your best not to take her rollercoaster emotions personally. The hormones surging through your partner's body can make a loving caress feel like sandpaper one minute, while the same touch a few hours later may lead to some of the hottest sex of your relationship. Trying to figure out when and where to be affectionate with your partner is arguably the most frustrating job of the expectant father. As with communication, your saving grace will be emotional flexibility.

That said, there is nothing in the procreation rule book that says men must relinquish all needs during pregnancy. It is important and necessary for you to merge your ability to communicate with your desire to be intimate with your partner. Explain that you want to hold, kiss, touch, and nuzzle her because you are attracted to her. Tell her how you are drawn to her changing body (but make sure you mean it!) and that you miss being affectionate. You will be surprised how many layers of stress can be melted away by warming her with your words first. Nine times out of 10, your genuine attempt to connect will be met with the physical intimacy you desired in the first place.

Changing the way you communicate and are affectionate with your partner during pregnancy inevitably leads your relationship to a much different place from where it started. Some fathers mourn this change. This is natural—it is likely that the early years of your relationship, or "the good old days," as some couples joke, were among the happiest of your whole life. Embracing a new version of your relationship is challenging and will take time. It can help to get support from someone other than your partner. Talking to other soon-to-be or new dads will help to normalize your feelings, as it will become immediately clear that you are all feeling similar things. Discussing the trouble you are having coping with pregnancy should not make you feel disloyal to your partner, or weak. It should be looked on as a tool to help you accept the new ways in which you and your partner relate to each other.

Finally, know that you are not alone in missing the way it used to be—study after study shows that most men struggle with a type of grief over their changing relationship during pregnancy. Taking time to acknowledge your feelings of loss permits you to enjoy your relationship on a spectrum and allow your identity as a couple to grow.

After this transition is overcome, many couples discover that pregnancy is a bridge that brings them closer together. The work put in to communicating better and trying to understand the other's pregnancy experience illustrates your commitment and dedication to each other. The knowledge that you both contributed to the life growing inside of mom is also a powerful bond. Though you will each play different roles throughout the course of parenthood, let yourselves be united by the knowledge that everything you know as parents, you will learn together.

SEX WITH A PREGNANT PARTNER

One of the earliest changes couples experience during pregnancy is a change in their sexual routine. It starts soon after deciding it is time to conceive. This is when intercourse becomes less about pleasure and more about the function of procreation. Changes continue throughout pregnancy. Once conception occurs, for example, you may become sex-crazed by your confirmed virility. Indeed, most men never discuss a fear they almost all share—the potential that they are "shooting blanks." Testosterone and pride aside, men often have a lingering doubt that they are, in fact, sterile. Therefore, learning that your sperm are champions capable of creating life can send your libido into overdrive! Further into pregnancy you may be turned on or off by your partner's changing body, and at some point find yourself afraid to have sex for fear of harming your baby with penetration (they say that's where dimples come from...). All of these reactions are completely normal and experienced by nearly all dads-to-be at some point. How deeply these shifts in perception affect your sex life, however, is up to you.

Unfortunately, your partner's libido may not always match yours— especially in the first few months when morning sickness and fatigue take their toll. You can express your sexual interest and attraction to her at this point, but respect her need for space. If she is simply not interested in having sex, give her time. She will come around when she feels better. In the meantime, feel free to masturbate as often as you like—without guilt—to take the "edge" off.

Of course, some men have little time for masturbation during pregnancy, because their partner feels very sexy and wants to make love one or more times a day. This usually happens during the first trimester when hormones surge through her body. Her appetite for sex may continue throughout pregnancy if she embraces her voluptuousness and wants to share her new curves with you.

However, problems may arise if one or both of you is turned off or repulsed by her weight gain. Indeed, gaining weight during pregnancy is a sensitive issue for women, and in some cases, for men, too. You may find your partner's widening hips and fuller breasts irresistible—or a complete turn-off. It depends on your personal aesthetics and what you love about your partner's body. But if you are not attracted to her, never ever tell her! Remember, you contributed to conception, and therefore to the changes in her body. Remember that you made a significant contribution in her getting to this point, so it is not fair to make her feel badly about her size. Instead, focus on connecting emotionally and know that she will get back to (or close to) her normal size again some day. For now, your job is to make her feel beautiful, secure, and loved.

Yet even the most secure and loving couples can still have issues with sex during pregnancy. A few reasons for this are the fear of damaging the fetus through penetration, piercing the amniotic sac, and causing preterm labor through orgasm. Though most men and women have these fears, they are unfounded in normal pregnancies. First, the fetus cannot be harmed by the penis during intercourse because it is protected by 2 membranes called the amnion and the chorion. These membranes fill with fluids to create the amniotic sac. This cushy home protects baby from both injury and infection. The amniotic sac is strong, buoyant, and flexible, so your penis will not pierce through its membranes.

What to Expect . . . . 🦆

And finally, the risk of an orgasm inducing early labor in normal pregnancies is nil. The contractions experienced after an orgasm are slight and normal and will not cause your partner's cervix to dilate or efface. However, if your partner has a high-risk pregnancy, your doctor will advise whether sex and orgasms are safe for mom and baby. But otherwise, sex is natural and pleasurable for pregnant couples who keep the lines of communication open.

SOCIAL LIFE

Pregnancy is a time of growth and change—physically and emotionally—for both you and your partner. Thus, each component of your life is affected as you experience the metamorphosis from couple into parents. The affects of pregnancy on your social life will depend on your partner's health, how often you go out now, and what your travel habits are. Though pregnancy does not have to destroy your social life, expect for it to be radically altered. Couples who go out on the town every other night will have some big social changes to make; couples who are already homebodies will have an easier transition to parenthood.

To figure out how parenthood is likely to affect your social life, take a few minutes to evaluate how you and your partner socialize. Let the following questions help you:
How many times a week do you go out as a couple? If you are used to going out more than twice a week, you are in for a rude awakening! One of the earliest and most persistent pregnancy symptoms is fatigue, which is also the primary reason your partner will probably not feel like socializing for much of her pregnancy. She will likely be too tired to go out more than once a week, and there may be weeks where she does not want to go out at all.

Do you usually go out for drinks and dinner? Happy hours are no longer happy for your nauseous partner. She obviously should not drink alcohol, smoke cigarettes, be exposed to secondhand smoke, or be on her feet for too long. This crosses most bars off the list of places that are fun for her to hang out in during pregnancy. In addition, she may want to skip restaurants until her stomach settles, which will be sometime around the fourteenth week of pregnancy. Wafting smells can be overwhelming and lead to several trips to the bathroom to throw up.

Is the late show your preferred show time? Timing is everything when it comes to socializing with your pregnant partner. Since most expectant mothers are ready for bed by 9 or 10 p.m., the late show is pretty much out of the question for awhile. If you are a movie lover, you may have to become matinee moviegoers. If she does feel like venturing out to the theater, bring along a cushion. She will appreciate the extra padding, since, as pregnancy progresses, it becomes difficult to sit for long stretches (the baby puts pressure on the tailbone, which can be quite painful). So, save the three-hour films for after she has the baby and stick to movies that are 90 minutes or less.

How often do you go out alone with the guys? If you are on a bowling team, in a band, and play poker every week, you should expect to drop at least one of these hobbies. Though it is important to carve out time for your individual needs, remember that your partner is limited by how she feels, and thus does not enjoy the same freedoms as you. Therefore, cutting activities back to one night a week is an act of solidarity your partner will appreciate and remember.

How much do you drink or smoke? Having a few drinks with friends now and then is fine, but you'll want to reduce your alcohol consumption and refrain from drinking a lot around your partner. Above all, quit smoking before your son or daughter is born. Limiting or giving up these vices reduces stress for your partner, prevents alcohol-infused arguments, avoids exposing your baby to secondhand smoke, and keeps temptation to drink or smoke at bay. Plus, men who adopt "the pregnancy lifestyle" in solidarity with their wives report feeling more connected to them throughout the pregnancy.

Do you and your partner like to travel frequently? Travel during normal pregnancies is safe and can be a wonderful bonding experience for you and your spouse. The second trimester tends to be the most agreeable time for car and air travel since morning sickness has usually subsided. If you must travel late in pregnancy, check with both your OB-GYN and your airline. Many carriers will not allow women to travel within a few weeks of their due date because of the risk of going into preterm labor and delivering on the plane! If you must travel any time during the third trimester, plan ahead by finding a local doctor and knowing the location of the closest hospital.

Depending on how you answered the above, your social life may or may not be impacted during pregnancy. It depends what you are used to doing, when, and with whom. And as with all of the other ways in which your life shifts around during pregnancy, your attitude about your changing social life is the key to your level of satisfaction.

BALANCING WORK AND HOME

Pregnancy is a time of transition that allows you to prepare for the big changes that occur once baby is born. Use these months wisely to figure out how you will balance your work schedule and home life after your child is born. For men with an 8-to-5 job this will be easier than for those who are required to put in overtime and travel.

In either case, your boss will appreciate your forward-thinking and candid expectations of how your role as employee may change after becoming a father.

To ascertain how hard you will have to work to achieve balance, consider the following:

How many hours do you currently work per week? If you are a lawyer who bills 80-plus hours a week, you are going to have a much different version of "cutting back" than the guy who clocks in to his office at 8 a.m. and is home by 5 p.m. No matter what your schedule is, be realistic about how much you can work while still leaving time to have a family. This is especially true in the first few weeks when mom is still recovering from delivery and initial bonding is happening with baby. Even beyond these first weeks, it is important to your child's development to have his father present. So take a hard look at your schedule. If you need to cut back, there are ways to do so without compromising your position in your company. Ask to work flexible hours, or to put in "4-10s"—that is, to work 10 hours 4 days a week, and take Fridays off. If these options are not possible and you cannot cut your hours, you may have to consider switching to a less time-consuming job.

Does your job require you to socialize with coworkers or clients? If your job requires you to spend several nights a week wining and dining clients or coworkers, talk to your boss about cutting back for awhile. Explain you would like to spend more time at home helping your partner. Offer to spend lunches or breakfasts with clients, or volunteer to train someone to take your place at these social events.

Do you have to travel for your job? If your job has you on the go, ask your boss to let you stay put for the last 4 weeks of pregnancy. During this time you will likely be finishing up childbirth classes, getting the house ready, and tending to your about-to-pop partner. The most important reason to be on home turf those last few weeks is if your baby comes early—you don't want to miss this life-altering moment because you were stuck in a hotel across the country! Offer to switch duties with a coworker or to do a different job until after your child is born. Your boss will appreciate your efforts to problem-solve and your desire to remain a team player.

Do you bring work home more than twice a week? Sometimes there simply are not enough hours in the day to get everything done. Increasingly, it is necessary to bring work home to finish a project or prep for the next one. This is often an acceptable reality for many childless couples. But as you prepare for fatherhood, you will want to start leaving work at work and making home about your family. If you have a good reputation and are productive during the day, speak to your boss about shifting some of your responsibilities to an assistant.

Do you keep commitments outside of work? Consider how many times you have agreed to meet your partner for dinner only to call and say, "Something came up at work." When it was just you two, this was probably not a point of contention. But once you become a father, keeping promises is important to building a strong family. Start reducing the number of nights you are kept away from home because of work. This helps your partner know you are committed to your new family and also helps coworkers shift their perception of you as "the guy you can always give more work to," to "the guy who is starting a family."

By now, you have hopefully developed a plan for how to integrate your life as an employee with your life as a father. If you conduct yourself with honesty, integrity, and continue to do high-quality work, chances are your boss will view you as irreplaceable and want to accommodate your new situation.

TAKING TIME OFF FROM WORK

When it comes to paid paternity leave, the United States falls short of most other countries. For example, Norway allows new fathers to take 35 weeks of leave with 100 percent pay (though time off is shared with mom's leave) or 45 weeks at 80 percent pay. Moreover, dads in Norway are required to take at least 6 weeks off; otherwise they forfeit the more generous paternity leave options. Sweden also has an impressive paternity program in place. New dads can take off up to 18 months (also shared with mom's leave) after baby is born and still earn 80 percent of their salary. The Swedish government actually requires that the "minority" caregiver, which is usually the father, take 3 months of paid leave to bond with baby. These nations' paternity leave programs are impressive testaments to how important they consider the father-child bond to be.

The United States, in contrast, does not offer federal paid leave for either parent. What is offered, however, is unpaid leave under the Family Medical Leave Act (FMLA) of 1993.

The FMLA can be confusing as there are many rules involved, and it covers more than just maternity and paternity leave. However, when used for childbirth or adoption, the FMLA offers unpaid leave with job protection and uninterrupted medical benefits to new parents for up to 12 weeks within the first year after the birth or adoption of a child.

What to Expect · · · · · · · · · ·

FMLA breaks down as follows:

- FMLA provides eligible employees with up to 12 weeks unpaid leave any time during the first 12 months after the birth or adoption of a child.

- Eligible employees must have been employed by their company or a federal, state, or local government agency for at least 12 months, though not necessarily consecutively.

- Eligible employees must have worked at least 1,250 hours for the company.

- The employer must have 50 or more employees within 75 miles of the worksite.

- FMLA does not have to be taken in consecutive weeks. It can be used intermittently throughout the first year of child's life. Check with your employer, however, because many companies require leave be taken in blocks of 2 weeks or more.

- Benefits remain intact, but the employee must continue to pay his portion while on leave.

- The employee has a right to return to the same salary, title, and benefits when leave is completed.

- The employee must apply for leave 30 days in advance of event or the employer may deny the request for time off.

- The employer may require certification from hospital or medical professionals.

- If both you and your partner work for the same company you cannot each take 12 weeks off—instead you must split the time, unless mom has serious health problems.

- Those with salaries in the top 10 percent of the company pay scale whose absence for 12 weeks would cause "substantial and grievous economic injury" to the company may not be eligible for FMLA leave.

- FMLA leave can be taken before birth for prenatal care, health problems, and preparing for baby.

Considering its limitations, you may not be surprised to learn that 78 percent of parents do not participate in FMLA. And though FMLA does have its benefits, relying on other programs, such as state-funded paid leave programs, is necessary for most dads. Some states, such as New Jersey and California, do offer paid programs. New Jersey's Family Leave Insurance and the California Paid Family Leave Program are state-funded by employees who pay into them through either Social Security Disability (SDI) or other state-sponsored insurance plans. In general, participants are entitled to up to 6 weeks leave and earn between 55 and 66 percent of their salary. There is a maximum amount per week, however, so check with your state to find out what it is when applying for benefits. States such as Arizona, Massachusetts, Minnesota, Pennsylvania, and New York are reviewing family leave bills, so if you live in one of these states, keep checking for updates.

In addition to state and federal leave, you should also save up vacation and sick time to use before and after baby comes. For many new dads, the best way to approach taking time off is to combine all of these options. Like with other work-related issues, the best approach to paternity leave is to give your employer plenty of notice and to communicate your needs. You may also want to consider working part-time, flex hours, or asking to work from home. Your boss is sure to appreciate your effort to stay connected to the office and value your commitment to both your job and your family.

RELIGIOUS ISSUES

Having a baby changes everything about your life—including how you feel about religion. Thus, even if you and your partner are not currently affiliated with a place of worship, do not be surprised if pregnancy causes one or both of you to revisit your childhood doctrines. Or, you may decide to abandon the religious traditions of your youth and raise your kids without or with a new religion. It is also common to be completely unsure about how religion should fit in your child's life. According to a poll by the American Religious Identification Survey (ARIS), approximately 81 percent of Americans identify with a specific religion while 16 percent reported abandoning religion all together. Meanwhile, a USA Today/Gallup poll found about 50 percent of Americans feel "alienated" by their religion, with 33 percent reporting they are "spiritual but not religious." This mixed data seems to reflect the changing landscape of religion in America, so it makes sense that you, too, may feel ambiguous about the issue.

There are certain areas in which religious guidance is comforting and helpful, even to those who are non-practicing. Decisions about circumcision, baptism, child care, and schooling are made easier for those with spiritual rules to guide them. Indeed, following the traditions of your congregation takes much of the guesswork out of otherwise difficult decisions. In addition, religious institutions are often community-based with generations of families together in one house of worship. This familiarity breeds family-like kinship and often provides valuable resources such as daycare.

In addition, organized religion also offers many structured activities designed to instill camaraderie, community responsibility, and integrity in both kids and adults. A recent Mississippi State

University study found that children who were raised with religion by parents who discussed their faith had better self-control, social skills, and ability to learn than kids whose parents were not religious. Researchers found, though, that necessary to the children's success were parents who held open discussions about faith and lived according to their beliefs. This shows that religion is not the sole indicator of raising a successful child but, rather, having parents who talk openly about faith-based issues. If religion is not your cup of tea, hold off on discussing it with your partner until after your baby is born. Trying to sort out such a weighty topic under the stress of pregnancy can lead to arguments.

One way to honor both partners when they differ on religion is to make a list of the values you want your child to grow up with. Chances are your lists will be close or identical. After discussing approaches for how to instill these values in your child, consider whether religion can help guide you. In turn, your partner may agree to have religious discussions when your child is old enough to participate in them. When you respect each other's feelings about religion, you set the precedent for how it will be discussed with your child later.

"A new baby is like the beginning of all things—wonder, hope, a dream of possibilities."
~ Eda J. Le Shan

Notes . . . .

Pregnancy!

CONGRATULATIONS! Your partner is pregnant. Even though you may have planned this, you are probably in shock nonetheless. If so, you are not alone. Deep down, many couples cannot imagine actually becoming pregnant, even though it is what they want most. Thinking about all of the decisions that must be made over the next 10 months can be overwhelming. This book will help guide you in the whirlwind that is pregnancy by breaking all of the information down into months. Before you delve into what's happening with mom and baby's development, some early decisions must be made. Use the following section to help you navigate through the early days—and beyond—of pregnancy.

A POSITIVE TEST

Waking one morning to your partner waving a pregnancy test wand and yelling, "We're pregnant!" may have your head spinning. You have been working hard to conceive, but now that you have done it you are not quite sure how it happened. Of course, you took sex education in high school, but now that you are actually faced with fatherhood, you cannot recall a single detail about how conception occurs beyond "sperm fertilizes egg." This is a perfectly normal reaction and happens to both expectant moms and dads alike. Re-learning how conception works, however, is both interesting and

Pregnancy! . . . .

necessary for making healthy decisions during this critical time of your baby's development.

Conception occurs when circumstances are just right during intercourse. Sperm works its way up into the fallopian tubes and is met by a mature egg. Though you release up to one billion sperm with each ejaculation, it only takes one sperm to penetrate the egg.

After getting inside the egg, the lucky sperm then creates a protective coating that prevents other sperm from penetrating it. At this moment of fertilization your child's entire genetic code is determined, including its hair and eye color, facial features, and sex. Each parent provides 23 chromosomes, but dad determines the baby's gender. Mom (XX) provides the X chromosome and dad (XY) either an X or Y. Delivery of an X chromosome means you can expect a daughter (XX), and if you supply a Y you have a son (XY) on the way.

After fertilization occurs, the egg and sperm form a single cell organism called a zygote. Within 12 hours, the zygote begins to quickly divide into many cells. It continues to double its size every 12 hours!

The zygote stays in the widest part of the fallopian tube for about 3 days before traveling toward the uterus for implantation. By the time it reaches the uterus, it is made up of about 500 cells and is called a blastocyst. The inner area of the blastocyst is fluid-filled. This fluid is what will eventually develop into your baby and the amniotic sac. The cells surrounding this cavity are called the trophoblast. This will later become the placenta, which will be your baby's "life raft." The blastocyst will embed itself in your partner's uterine lining, or endometrium.

. . . . Pregnancy!

Around this time, mom's body starts to produce the human chorionic gonadotropin (hCG) hormone. HCG supports her pregnancy and can be detected in her urine some time between 1 and 2 weeks after conception by an at-home pregnancy test. In fact, some home pregnancy tests can detect hCG in the urine as early as six days after fertilization. HCG levels will double every few days during the first 10 to 12 weeks of her pregnancy.

Though your partner may not test positive until several weeks—or even a month—after her last period, doctors consider a pregnancy to begin on the first day of her last menstrual period (LMP). However, until a fertilized egg implants itself in your partner's uterus, she is not actually pregnant. Doctors calculate pregnancy this way for the convenience of time of reference, but conception does not actually occur until about two weeks later. Therefore, pregnancy lasts 40 weeks according to the LMP timeline, whereas actual pregnancy is 38 weeks. This can seem a bit confusing at first, but you will get used to calculating pregnancy in terms of weeks once it gets rolling and your partner has monthly doctor's visits.

Far before you set foot into the OB-GYN's office, your partner's uterine lining has begun to thicken in order to become habitable for implantation. Implantation occurs when the endometrium is thick enough to accept the blastocyst. Approximately 12 days after fertilization, the blastocyst sticks to the endometrium and releases enzymes that allow it to embed itself in the uterine wall. This microscopic gesture is akin to a space shuttle landing on the moon—and every bit as momentous.

It is common for women to experience some bleeding or to feel a pinching sensation as the blastocyst works it way into the endometrium. As implantation continues, her body produces high levels of progesterone and estrogen. These hormones will be

Pregnancy! . . . .

responsible for the many changes to her breasts, cervix, and uterus over the next several months.

After implantation, your little ball of cells becomes an embryo and continues to burrow deeper into the endometrium. The embryo is tiny—a mere .006 inches long! Even though it is still very early in the pregnancy, your embryo's brain, spinal cord, and heart have already started to develop. It is also busy building what will become the amniotic sac, which will cushion and protect your baby as it grows. The amniotic bag will eventually house your son or daughter. It will contain amniotic fluid, which is mostly made up of water.

The amniotic sac's main job is to protect your baby when he is jostled about as your partner goes about her daily routine. The surface of the amniotic sac is tough. By the 34th week, it is big enough to house both your baby and a full quart of amniotic fluid. There are several amazing biological tools that will help your baby develop properly, and the amniotic sac is definitely one of them.

Once embedded in the endometrium, the embryo attaches itself to the uterine wall by connective tissues called villi (anchoring stems). Villi are responsible for fusing the embryonic cells to the endometrium and for allowing maximum surface-area contact between the embryo and uterus. Mom's blood reaches the embryo through villi to nourish your growing baby.

By the second week after fertilization, the embryo is just 1/25 of an inch long. Still, it is hard at work organizing its layered cells for development. The outer layer, or ectoderm, will produce your baby's neural tube from which his spine and brain will form. The middle layer, or mesoderm, is the setting for the growth of your baby's heart and circulatory system, as well as reproductive organs and bones. The inner layer, or endoderm, will produce your baby's intestines, lungs, and bladder.

Meanwhile, pregnancy hormones have your partner's body working overtime to create a sustainable environment for your baby to flourish in. As a result, she may be exhausted and experience mood swings. It is around this time that mom experiences hormone-related symptoms, such as sore breasts and fatigue. In fact, sore breasts are often the first clue that pregnancy has occurred.

PRENATAL CARE

Getting good prenatal care is one of the most important ways to ensure a healthy pregnancy. In fact, the U.S. Department of Health and Human Services reports that mothers who go without prenatal care are 3 times more likely to have low-birth-weight babies—a leading cause of infant mortality. Therefore, to have the healthiest pregnancy—and child—possible, you and your partner must work as a team to ensure she has access to excellent prenatal care.

The first major decision is choosing the right doctor or midwife to monitor mom and baby. There are several factors to consider before selecting a healthcare provider, including types of providers, bedside manner, finances and insurance, desired birth location, and mom's health.

TYPES OF PROVIDERS

Family Physician (FP): Your family physician may or may not follow pregnancy and delivery, but if your partner is attached to him or her, it can't hurt to ask. FP prenatal care is reserved for low-risk, normal pregnancies. Most people who choose their FP as their prenatal doctor live in rural areas or have a long history

Pregnancy! . . . .

with the doctor. An FP follows usual medical protocol and will use medication and intervention if deemed necessary. Insurance will cover FP care and delivery usually takes place in a hospital, unless your family lives in an extremely remote location.

Obstetrician-Gynecologist (OB-GYN): Not all gynecologists work with pregnant women, but OB-GYNs specialize in female reproductive health and pregnancy. They can usually monitor normal to complicated pregnancies (and everything in between). Still, an OB-GYN may refer your partner out to a perinatologist or maternal-fetal specialist if she has severe complications. An OB-GYN can perform Cesarean deliveries as well as administer medications and perform other interventions, such as labor induction or prevention. An OB-GYN delivers babies in a hospital and follows medical protocol, though she should respect your family's birth plan. Insurance covers OB-GYN care, but the level of coverage depends on your plan.

Certified Nurse-Midwife (CNM): A CNM has a bachelor's (or higher) degree and is licensed by the American College of Nurse-Midwives. A CNM is educated in both nursing and midwifery and must pass a certification exam. She is able to do routine exams, pap smears, prescribe birth control, and provide prenatal care. A CNM will attend births that occur in the home, hospital, or birthing center. CNMs support natural birthing methods and are less likely to push for medical interventions. Use of a CNM is usually limited to low-risk pregnancies, but should complications develop, she will have an OB-GYN on-call as well. Insurance coverage varies, but at the time of this printing more than 25 states required HMO and other plans to cover prenatal care given by a CNM. And all 50 states require Medicaid coverage for CNM care. Other types of midwives include Certified Professional Midwife (CPM), Direct-

Entry Midwife (DEM), Certified Midwife (CM), and Lay Midwife (LM). For more information on midwives visit www.midwife.org or www.narm.org.

Once your family decides on the type of provider to use, it is time to select one to work with throughout the pregnancy. It is helpful to interview a few doctors or midwives to determine which one meets your partner's needs. If possible, go with her and have a list of questions ready to facilitate the interview process.

The following list of considerations and questions can help gauge if he or she is the right person for the job:

- How helpful is the front desk and nursing staff?
- How long has the doctor been in practice?
- How many babies has she delivered in her career?
- How much time is allotted for prenatal visits?
- What prenatal tests does he recommend?
- What if your partner refuses a particular test she recommends?
- Is he equipped to handle high-risk pregnancies?
- Does she explain difficult concepts in a way you can understand?
- Do you have his undivided attention?
- Does your partner seem relaxed in her presence?
- How accessible is she?
- What is the turnaround time on phone calls?
- How large is his practice?
- Who provides back-up when she is out of town?
- Will you always see the same doctor/midwife?
- Is the location of the birth flexible?
- At which hospital or birthing center does he usually deliver babies?
- Does she accept your insurance?
- What fees are not covered by insurance?

Pregnancy! . . . .

- How does he feel about breast-feeding?
- When should you call during labor?
- Will she honor your birth plan (barring emergencies)?
- How often does he use medical interventions?
- Will she honor your partner's desire to avoid pain medication during labor and delivery?
- Will he honor your partner's desire for quick pain relief during labor and delivery?
- How many Cesarean births has she done?
- How often does he induce labor?
- How often does she use delivery tools, such as forceps or the vacuum?
- Will he allow a doula, friends, and/or family to be present at the birth?
- How often does she perform episiotomies?
- Does he perform circumcisions?
- Does she answer questions to your satisfaction?
- Does he take your concerns seriously, or do you feel like a pest?
- Do both you and your partner feel comfortable with this person?

After you select your healthcare provider, your first prenatal exam will be scheduled for when your partner is around 8 weeks pregnant. Each appointment thereafter will be once a month until the third trimester. At the end of the pregnancy, the provider will see your partner once every two weeks and finally once a week until delivery.

You should attend as many of these prenatal visits as possible. This is one way for you to connect with the pregnancy and to be part of the action. In addition, your presence will be comforting to your partner as well as establish you as an interested parent.

This will come in handy if you must call the doctor's office with a routine question or during an emergency. Besides, being an active participant in your child's prenatal care is good practice for true fatherhood.

Another benefit of attending prenatal visits is getting a first-hand look at what your partner goes through each month. During each visit she will have her weight and blood pressure checked. She will provide a urine sample to be tested for the hCG hormone, protein, and sugar. The doctor will also measure the size of her uterus by external and/or internal examination and check her face and ankles for swelling. You should use each appointment as an opportunity to ask questions and discuss issues that may be troubling you, such as upcoming prenatal tests.

Prenatal testing is routine in the United States, and there are many different kinds of tests you'll need to learn about. Some tests are basic and routine, while others are believed to pose a possible risk to your child. Each visit to the doctor should yield some discussion of what tests are coming up and whether they are necessary. Most tests have a success window, meaning if they are not done during a certain time frame they will not produce the desired results.

Later on in this book we will get further into the details of prenatal testing, but below is a cursory glance at the most commonly offered tests and when they occur:
Pregnancy test: usually offered between 6 and 21 days of fertilization

Blood tests: first prenatal visit and as needed throughout pregnancy

Pap smear: first visit

Pregnancy! . . . .

Urine sample: each visit

Chorionic Villus Sampling (CVS): between 10 and 12 weeks of pregnancy

Maternal Blood Screening/Triple Screen/Quadruple Screen: usually done between 15 and 20 weeks of pregnancy

Amniocentesis: usually done between 15 and 20 weeks of pregnancy, but after the Maternal Blood Screening/Triple Screen/Quadruple Screen

Ultrasound: at 18 to 20 weeks of pregnancy and then as needed

Percutaneous Umbilical Blood Sampling (PUBS): after 18 weeks of pregnancy

Glucose Screening: done between 24 and 28 weeks of pregnancy

Nonstress Test: can be done any time after 26 or 28 weeks

Strep B swab: between 35 and 37 weeks

Contraction Stress Test: As needed, if the doctor is concerned about how baby will respond to contractions

In addition to attending monthly appointments, you can help your partner maintain a healthy diet, positive attitude, and regular exercise routine, each of which are an important part of good prenatal care. The support you lend your partner in these areas during this time is invaluable. Make yourself available to her. Eat better, quit smoking, and drink less. And of course, offer lots of encouragement. This support will benefit her health and that of your baby.

SHARING THE NEWS

Finding out your partner is pregnant may have you hanging from the rafters with a megaphone ready to shout to the world that you are going to be a father. But before making the big announcement, there are some important things to consider. You and your partner will want to be clear on when you share the news, how you do it, and who gets to know first. Be aware of what the consequences of sharing too early (or too late) might be. Above all, sharing your great news with anyone outside of your relationship is a joint decision that should be carefully considered and agreed upon by both of you.

When deciding who and when to tell, do not be surprised if your partner has a very short list in the beginning. Many women are terrified of miscarrying. As a result, they want to avoid having to potentially tell a bunch of people they lost the baby in the event this tragedy occurs. Even though miscarriage is not usually a woman's fault, many women take it very personally and even as a sign that they did something wrong to lose the baby. Having to tell others they are no longer pregnant, therefore, is not only emotionally upsetting for them but raises fears that others will judge them as being a bad mother.

For this reason, most couples wait until the beginning of the second trimester to tell the news to those outside of their immediate circle. Given that 10 to 25 percent of all pregnancies are spontaneously aborted during the first 20 weeks of implantation—with most occurring before 13 weeks—it makes sense to wait. And the odds of losing the baby increases with the age of the mother. Women 30 to 45 years old have a 20 to 35 percent of miscarriage, while women 45 and older face a 50 percent chance of losing the pregnancy.

But fear of miscarriage is not the only reason couples wait to share the news. Another reason is to preserve your work situation until you are able to get a handle on your company's family leave policy. Waiting gives you time to feel out your boss's attitude toward paternity leave and evaluate your coworkers' willingness to help out around the office. Many dads-to-be prefer to sniff out what the family vibe is at their jobs before singling themselves out as a father. The fact is, some professions view paternity leave as unnecessary. In some cases, even discussing leave can open you up to scrutiny that leads to missed promotions and/or raises. Though this is rare and illegal, it does happen. Therefore, saving your news for when you are confident it will be well-received can help insulate you against possible challenges to your career.

Another reason to keep the news close to the vest is to limit the number of well-wishing-advice-givers. These folks are family, friends, coworkers, and acquaintances who feel obliged to share the best and worst stories regarding pregnancy and birth. No one quite knows why, but some people are compelled to tell expectant parents about a cousin who spent 27 hours in labor only to end up having a Cesarean delivery during a black out. You cannot avoid these folks entirely, but waiting until the second trimester when you are less worried about losing the baby can limit the extent to which their stories influence you.

The flipside of the horror story is the, "I know how to have the easiest pregnancy (or birth) ever" person. This type of tale feels less like an assault and more like an indictment. It often starts out with innocent yet irritating suggestions, such as, "Make sure your wife eats lots of asparagus! I ate nothing but asparagus and it completely eliminated my nausea!" or, "Tell your partner to deliver at Hospital X. They're the only ones in town who know anything about delivering babies!"

Although it is usually well-meaning, beneath the advice lies the judgment that you are doing it "wrong" if you do not follow their "expert" advice. This will be more difficult for your partner to manage, since she will be on the receiving end of most of these interactions. But you can help shield her by deflecting these kinds of comments. Make a joke and follow it up with a swift exit.

So, keeping the pregnancy under wraps for awhile limits your exposure to those who are dying to share best-and-worst case scenarios. However, there are benefits to sharing the news with your close circle right away. They include:

- Early support from loved ones
- The ability to be emotional in front of people who know you well
- Early offers of help to get things done
- Family advice and secrets about how to manage pregnancy symptoms
- Suggestions for doctors, hospitals, etc.
- Tips and advice for bargain hunting
- Avoid hurting the feelings of parents or close friends
- Connecting with friends who are pregnant or who have children
- Your partner can begin getting pampered immediately
- Built-in support system should something go wrong with the pregnancy

In sum, there are many advantages and disadvantages to sharing the news early with others. You and your partner will have to decide what is best for your family. Whenever you decide to tell the people in your life, make sure you agree with your partner on how it is done. Some couples find it important to be together and make a formal announcement. Others prefer to send out an email or note with the news. And some quietly and privately tell whomever they feel like it when the moment strikes.

Establishing rules for sharing the news can prevent misunder-standings between you and your partner and ensures that your monumental announcement is delivered as you wish it to be. If this is to be your only child, you will only get one chance to tell others about it. Consider it to be like the other important moments of your relationship that you wanted to go a certain way: the day you got engaged, the day you were married, and other events you wanted to be just right.

NAMING YOUR CHILD

Choosing a name for your child is one of the most important decisions you will make as a parent. Some couples have always known what they would name a son or daughter, and so for them, the decision is already made. But for most people there are many considerations, such as family input, religion, how it sounds when said aloud, the tease-factor, and whether you will call your baby by his full name or use a nickname. In addition, parents must decide whether to stick with an early name choice or choose a few names and wait until baby is born to see which one fits.

Two of the larger forces at work when naming a child are family and religion. Some families expect to have the same name passed down for generations and bucking the system can be difficult and hurtful. Hopefully, your partner will be onboard if this is the case. But if not, talk to your family about using the name as your baby's middle name instead of first.

The same holds true for religious names. If you and your partner are not keen on naming your baby Mary, Moses, or Mohammed, consider saving the heavy-hitting name for your child's middle name, or use the first initial (for example, naming your daughter Margaret). In some traditions, it is common to name a child after the first initial of other relatives—this can help honor more relatives at once. For example, both your Grandfather Stanley and your Aunt Sarah can by honored by naming your child Simon. Though family members may get bent out of shape when they first hear the name you have chosen, it will not last. They will fall in line and call your baby whatever you want as long as they get to spend time with him!

Other issues to consider when selecting a name are how it sounds when spoken aloud and whether it sets your child up for teasing during school years. Indeed, some names look fine on paper but simply do not flow when said out loud. Other names look good, sound fine, but harbor the potential for cruel nicknames that invite merciless teasing later on. Also consider the spelling of your child's name. It may seem creative to spell your daughter's name Christeena, or Lorrie, but know that you are dooming her to a childhood without personalized keychains, t-shirts, and other such treasures that become priceless to children at a certain age. Finally, consider how "ethnic" a name you give your child. It is important to some couples that they give their child a cultural name that has meaning to them. But consider that such a name might be difficult for teachers and students to pronounce as your child progresses through school. The last thing you want is have the name you put so much thought into turn into a burden or an embarrassment for your child. You and your partner will have to consider all of these issues as you sift through potential names for your child.

As you share names with each other, avoid the urge to make fun of your partner's choices. If you set up a rivalry to find the "best" name, you will always be in opposition and never agree. Instead, each of you should write down your top 5 choices and exchange your lists. Spend time with each other's list before making any comments. Allow each other to cross off 2 or 3 names that you can't stand and agree to discuss the others. Also, it can help to talk about what you want in a name. What is important to you? Passing down a tradition? Religious context? Choosing a meaningful name from a movie or book that you and your partner both enjoyed? Establishing a few parameters may help narrow down your choices and keep the conversation civil.

Every year, certain names find favor among thousands of couples across the America. According to the Social Security Administration, in 2010 the top 10 names were:

Rank	Male name	Female name
1	Jacob	Emma
2	Michael	Isabella
3	Ethan	Emily
4	Joshua	Madison
5	Daniel	Ava
6	Alexander	Olivia
7	Anthony	Sophia
8	William	Abigail
9	Christopher	Elizabeth
10	Matthew	Chloe

You and your partner may get a laugh out of seeing that several of the names on your lists are among the most common in the country.

DAD: THE FAMILY AMBASSADOR

Pregnancy can bring out both the best and the worst in people's families. It often seems as though family members respond in one of two ways: they either want to help to the point of suffocating you and your partner, or relatives are so timid that it feels as if you are stranded on Pregnancy Island. Hopefully, you are lucky enough to be graced with relatives who fall somewhere in between these extremes. Familial support is extremely important both during pregnancy and once your baby is born. As author Jane Howard once put it, "Call it a clan, call it a network, call it a tribe, call it a family. Whatever you call it, whoever you are, you need one." That said, you and your partner must decide the level of involvement you will tolerate from grandparents, aunts, uncles, and other well-meaning relatives. And once decisions are made, such as who can visit the hospital, how long grandparents can stay with you after baby is born, and what the at-home visiting hours are, be prepared, as the father of the child, to become the enforcer of these rules.

Indeed, management of family members (and friends) is one job that definitely falls on dad. There are many reasons why you are better equipped to fend off intrusive relatives or enlist the help of absent ones. One is that during pregnancy mom is flooded with hormones that may backfire and cause her to give in to her pushy mother or be reluctant to ask for help from a distant mother-in-law. In addition, dads are usually better at taking an authoritative tone that relatives are less likely to argue with. Running interference between mom and family members will be especially important during labor and delivery and in the weeks immediately after your baby is born.

One of the first family decisions you and your partner should make is who will be permitted in the delivery room. It may sound too early to be thinking about that, but you would be amazed at how attached people get to the idea of being present during the birth—some relatives may even assume you will have them present even if you haven't asked, and will spend the duration of your wife's pregnancy imagining themselves in the room on birth day. The disappointment that results when they find out they won't be included is magnified by the amount of time they have been thinking they would be present. Therefore, it is in everyone's best interest to get delivery room attendance lists out of the way as early as possible.

Some women want their mothers or sisters present and some prefer it just be you and the medical staff. Whatever is decided, let the family know before the big day so there is no confusion. Tell relatives who are invited to the birth ahead of time that their attendance is conditional upon how smoothly labor and delivery progresses. Prepare them to be booted from the room if your partner changes her mind and thank them in advance for understanding. And do not be afraid to disappoint a grandparent or brother-in-law who was hoping to videotape your child's entry into this world by saying "No" to their request to be present.

Your job as family ambassador does not end there. Keeping people away from the hospital is a lot easier than it will be to keep them away once baby comes home. However, it is important to establish visiting hours—particularly during the first week when your family's immediate priority is bonding with your baby and sleeping when you can. During this time, your partner will be recovering from delivery and getting used to nursing. If she is comfortable with breast-feeding in front of people this may be less of an issue. However, she will certainly appreciate you fielding phone calls and sending drop-ins away until you are all ready to receive guests.

This may not sound like an ideal job, but it is crucial to your immediate family unit. Setting boundaries with both extended families also sets the precedent that you and your partner are in charge and capable of handling your new responsibilities as parents. Care should be taken when establishing ground rules, because your partner will need help once you go back to work.

Another area in which you can be of help is working with the grandparents (and other relatives who are willing to pitch in) to establish a "help schedule" for when you go back to work. On average, most men are initially home between 1 and 2 weeks, and then mom is left alone with a newborn. This can be overwhelming, especially if she is recovering from a C-section or is having issues with nursing. Therefore, setting up a schedule for grandmas, aunts, and friends to come do housework, cook, or entertain baby while mom naps will go a long way toward reassuring your partner that she will be OK without you.

But long before your baby arrives there is work to be done for the family ambassador. Thinking of yourself in this role early in pregnancy shows your partner that she can depend on you to step up. Establishing yourself as the go-between from the get-go will make your life easier later in the pregnancy—and beyond— because you will have already laid the groundwork that you are a father who does, in fact, know what is best for his family.

YOUR MIXED EMOTIONS

Pregnancy is a time of mixed emotions for both partners, but fathers-to-be have a specific set of reactions that is unique to men. And since men are less likely to discuss these feelings with their partners, friends, or family, they tend to suffer in silence. This behavior allows pent-up emotions to turn into near-debilitating levels of stress. Indeed, the American Psychological Association (APA) conducted a 2007 Stress in America Survey that discovered 50 percent of men felt their stress had reached a critical level. In addition, men acknowledged that too much stress negatively affected their level of satisfaction with their lives. Since pregnancy is such a tumultuous time for most men, it is important to sift through your emotions and share them to prevent stress from accumulating.

The first step toward getting a handle on your emotions is to identify them. Feelings of joy, responsibility, pride, and fear can get mixed up in your emotional blender, and teasing them out can be difficult. But when you begin to analyze each distinct reaction and emotion, you begin to reduce your sense of powerlessness, alienation, and even guilt.

Two surprising yet common emotions felt by men during their partner's pregnancy are resentment and jealousy. Common reasons for feeling jealous or resentful include:

- Your partner's attention being shifted away from you toward the pregnancy
- Mom's immediate attachment to the pregnancy
- Your partner's role as "life raft" to baby
- Everyone's attention directed toward your partner
- Maternity leave versus paternity leave benefits
- Your role as provider
- Feeling ignored by the doctor or midwife
- Pregnancy used as a "get out of jail free" card for just about anything
- Financial burdens of having a baby
- Cutting down on (or eliminating) social drinking and smoking
- Limiting time with friends
- Taking care of a partner who is sick from pregnancy complications
- Diminished sex life

It can be difficult to share these feelings with your partner, so find a male friend or relative to confide in. Otherwise, you may end up feeling like an ugly person on the inside. Plus, sharing these thoughts with another man who has experienced them has redemptive qualities that relieve a guilty conscience.

It is also possible that while you are excited about having a baby, the idea to procreate was more your partner's than your own. Across the board, it is much more common for women to get "baby fever" than men. This is in part due to the increasingly loud ticking of their "biological clock," which men, since they can procreate longer than women, do not feel as acutely.

In fact, it is entirely probable that you would have continued enjoying your baby-free existence for a good many years to come. Maybe you feel reluctant to have to spend your extra money on a child instead of new tools, CDs, or gadgets for yourself. Maybe you are dreading having to keep the house extra neat, clean, and organized. Maybe, even, you are afraid that having a child officially marks the end of your own youth, something you are not entirely ready to relinquish. In fact, many men report that they don't think of themselves as being "old enough" to have a baby, even when they have more than surpassed the age of procreation.

Each of these are natural, understandable feelings that are shared by countless men. Take comfort in the fact that your fears are sure to pass once you hold your son or daughter in your arms for the first time. They will continue to diminish when you realize that having a child is not necessarily a grown-up prison sentence—in fact, as your child gets older, many men enjoy the chance to become a child again themselves. Playing baseball, thinking up Halloween costumes, and conducting kitchen-science experiments are just a few of the ways in which fatherhood has turned many men into boys once again.

Pregnancy! . . . .

But no matter what your negative emotions have been, it is more likely that you are feeling overwhelmed by positive feelings. Chances are you have been looking forward to becoming a father and have been working at conception with your partner for quite a while. Now that she is pregnant, your thoughts are turning to dreams of seeing your son graduate with honors or teaching your daughter to play guitar. You feel a flurry of excitement when you imagine how much fun you will have as a family and how your child is going to make you laugh harder than any movie you've ever watched or joke you've ever heard.

Feelings of joy, excitement, and pride may flood you when you least expect it. These can bring even the most stoic man to tears! This does not make you less of man, but rather makes you more of a father. Embrace these feelings and let them work their magic.

Common reasons for bursts of joy, excitement, and pride include:

- You are not sterile!
- You always wanted to be a father.
- You weren't sure you wanted to be a father until now.
- You helped create a human being.
- You are in awe of your partner's body.
- Feeling the baby kick for the first time.
- Seeing baby on an ultrasound
- Feeling closer to your partner
- Imagining your first trip as a dad to an amusement park or baseball game with your son or daughter
- Attending graduations and weddings
- Passing on your name
- Sharing your knowledge with your child
- Passing down family traditions

Of course, you will most often find yourself in a state of flux that includes some combination of fear and happiness. This is normal. Do not think you are losing your mind or your manhood. Becoming a father is a complex state of being that requires both lifestyle and emotional transitions that take time.

HOW TO HANDLE YOUR PARTNER'S EMOTIONS

Dealing with your own emotions is one thing, but handling your pregnant partner can feel a bit like turning the crank on a Jack-in-the-Box at times. You are going about your normal business when suddenly, "Whap!" A door opens and your partner has been replaced by a terrifying, screeching, crying, wobbling, bobble-head. It's OK to laugh! It's funny because it's true. Even pregnant women acknowledge their Jekyll-and-Hyde-like personalities. It is impossible not to notice the emotional changes that occur during pregnancy. Handling your partner's hormone fueled emotions takes patience, sensitivity, and a healthy sense of humor.

Thankfully, there are ways to troubleshoot your partner's emotional instability. The following suggestions may go a long way in preventing you from ending up at the wrong end of the pregnancy rifle:

If she is feeling irritable or displaying symptoms of PMS: Give her space. Don't point out her mood.

If she is weepy: Let her cry. Get her a tissue. Baby her a bit.

If she is exhausted: Do a few chores and keep the volume on the TV down so she can rest.

If she feels or looks unattractive: Tell her she looks great and exactly as she is supposed to at this stage in her life.

Pregnancy! . . . .

If she feels or looks fat: Never agree with her or point out her weight gain.

If she appears consumed by the pregnancy: Encourage outside interests and hobbies.

If she feels overwhelmed by responsibility: Share your feelings so she feels less alone.

If she is tired of feeling sick: Give her lots of praise and encouragement.

If she is terrified of giving birth: Assure her you are there every step of the way.

If she is afraid of being a bad mother: Tell her you're afraid of fatherhood, too, but that'll you support each other.

If she is concerned about going back to work: Let her know you'll figure it out together.

If she is nervous about breast-feeding: Remind her there are resources to help with nursing.

If she is inexplicably angry: Don't take it personally, and try not to get angry in response.

If she is bored with being pregnant: Remind her it is a temporary situation.

If she is worried about the baby's health: Share your fears and confidence about your healthy child.

If she is demanding or impatient: Exercise patience, and calmly ask that she respect that you are doing your best.

The way you handle your partner's emotions says a lot about who you will be as a father. Think about it. Kids are completely irrational and demanding. They want what they want when they want it. But you wouldn't storm off or ignore your child in the midst of an emotional crisis. Likewise, treat your partner with patience and kindness when she gets off-the-wall crazy. Deal with her firmly, yet sympathetically. Be fair and reasonable when she cannot be. Remind yourself that her tantrums, tears, and meltdowns are the result of hormones circulating in her body. In many ways, learning to manage your partner's extreme mood swings is nothing less than excellent practice for being a dad.

"The soul is healed by being with children."
~ Fyodor Dostoyevsky

Notes . . . .

Lunar Month

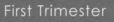

One

First Trimester

Lunar Month one . . . .

MONTHLY TO-DO LISTS

- ❏ Learn what foods trigger morning sickness and avoid eating them around your partner
- ❏ Learn what products have smells (such as soaps, deodorants, etc.) that trigger morning sickness and avoid using them around your partner
- ❏ Offer to walk or swim with your partner 2-3 times a week
- ❏ Expect your partner to have mood swings
- ❏ Encourage your partner to take prenatal vitamins
- ❏ Take the first shower so your partner can sleep in
- ❏ Anticipate your partner may have an increased or decreased sex drive
- ❏ Take over cleaning the litter box if you have a cat—mom should not be exposed to it
- ❏ Quit smoking
- ❏ Reduce alcohol consumption
- ❏ Check in to see how your partner is feeling daily

MY PERSONAL CHECKLIST:

- ❏ ....
- ❏ ....
- ❏ ....

MY HOPES FOR THIS MONTH:

....

....

....

....

....

....

....

What's Happening: Mom & Baby

LUNAR MONTH 1

First Trimester

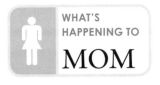

WHAT'S HAPPENING TO MOM

THIS FIRST MONTH of pregnancy encompasses conception, fertilization, and implantation. Each of these amazing processes are accompanied by symptoms. Since all women experience pregnancy differently, your partner may suffer a lot of symptoms this month, or she may have none.

Many of the first month's symptoms are similar to those of premenstrual syndrome (PMS). This means you can expect your partner to be irritable and moody. She may also have to urinate frequently, experience breast tenderness, be fatigued, and suffer from persistent nausea. Unlike PMS, however, the reasons for her condition are due to the rush of hormones that are released once fertilization and implantation occur. Symptoms may last a few weeks or come and go throughout the entire pregnancy.

While hormones wreak havoc on a woman's body throughout pregnancy, this is particularly true during the early stages. One of the earliest hormones released at this time is progesterone. Your partner's body produces this essential hormone when the fertilized egg successfully implants in the endometrium and she misses her next period. Progesterone has many jobs during pregnancy, including

MOM'S
Symptoms

- Fatigue
- Dizziness
- Nausea
- Heartburn
- Gas
- Breast tenderness
- Implantation staining and/ or cramping
- Frequent urination
- Irritability
- Mood swings
- Crying spells

suppressing her immune system so her body will not attack the embryo. Progesterone also prevents the uterus from contracting, and causes blood vessel growth in the endometrium.

Another heavy-hitting hormone is estrogen. Its main job at this stage is to build tissue by increasing the number and size of blood cells and vessels. This causes mom's breasts to enlarge as her ducts expand to make room for the milk that will later feed your baby. This "breast expansion project" may sound like a dream come true to you, but for your partner it can be the first painful side effect of pregnancy. Her breasts are likely to become very sore and tender. In fact, many women report this excessive breast soreness as their first clue they are pregnant.

Estrogen is also responsible for the thickening and stretching of your partner's womb, as well as for the increased blood flow to her uterus. This increases pressure on her bladder, which likely has her running to the bathroom several times a day. In addition, estrogen decreases the production of hydrochloric acid and pepsin in mom's digestive tract. As a result, her ability to digest fat is decreased, leading to upset stomach and nausea.

This month, your partner's body is also manufacturing high levels of the human chorionic gonadotropin (hCG) hormone. This is the hormone that is detected by pregnancy tests. This is why you should wait to take a test until around 3 to 4 weeks after your partner's last period. At this point, hCG levels should be high enough to get a positive reading from an at-home test. Another important function of hCG is that it causes the ovaries to continue to produce progesterone, which is necessary for sustaining the pregnancy. In fact, without hCG, your partner's body would stop producing progesterone and she would get her period.

Of course, all of these hormonal changes take their toll on your partner's body. She may be consistently fatigued and require additional rest to prevent frequent meltdowns. Try and think about her body during this period as being "under construction." It is transforming into a life-support system capable of sustaining both a woman and a baby for up to 42 weeks. The effects of these changes are unpredictable and come and go in waves, so your partner may feel out of control of her body and her emotions. On a typical day she might wake up feeling sick to her stomach and unrested. This may cause her to snap at you over breakfast, then call you at work, crying, apologetic, and terrified that she will not be able to survive 40 or so weeks of pregnancy. When she gets

ⓘ PREGNANCY FACT

Doctors consider a pregnancy to begin on the first day of your partner's last menstrual period (LMP). However, until a fertilized egg implants itself in the uterus, she isn't actually pregnant. Doctors calculate pregnancy this way for the convenience of time of reference, but you should understand that conception doesn't actually occur until about 2 weeks later. Therefore, pregnancy lasts 40 weeks according to the LMP timeline, whereas actual pregnancy is 38 weeks.

home from work she might crash on the couch for an hour only to wake feeling excited about the pregnancy. These ups and downs are to be expected and should even out sometime during the second trimester as hormones level off.

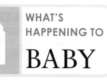

WHAT'S HAPPENING TO BABY

The first month of your baby's development is a critical and amazing time. By the end of the first 4 weeks she may be up to 1/3 of an inch long and have the earliest formations of her eyes, ears, nose, mouth, chin, and neck. In addition, her liver, gall bladder, arms, and legs will all start to develop. Perhaps most astonishing is that her heart will beat more than 100 times per minute by the end of the month! Therefore, it is crucial during this time that you support your partner's good health. It is in this earliest stage of development that baby is most susceptible to damage from harmful toxins, such as nicotine and alcohol.

Once fertilization occurs, things happen very quickly. The zygote, or fertilized egg, continues to divide—a process called mitosis. By the time your baby is born, she will be made up of more than 2 trillion cells! Inside each of these cells is a nucleus in which your baby's entire genetic code is contained. As mitosis generates more cells, identical copies of her DNA are made.

When the zygote is about 100 cells, it takes the shape of a sphere that surrounds a fluid-filled pocket. This fluid-filled area eventually develops into your baby and the amniotic sac. The cells around this area are called the trophoblast and will become the placenta.

Now called a blastocyst, your baby secretes enzymes that eat away at the endometrium to make a spot in which to embed itself. After implantation—which usually occurs around 12 to 14 days after fertilization—your baby becomes known as an embryo. The embryo is able to burrow deep into the lining of the uterus during the implantation process thanks to enzymes secreted during this stage.

After implanting, the embryo is connected to the endometrium by villi. Villi are connective tissues that fuse embryonic cells to the uterine wall. Nutrients from maternal blood reach the embryo through villi and provide nourishment until the placenta forms. Other important structures to develop this month are the yolk sac and amnion. These will house and feed the embryo. The yolk sac produces blood cells that nourish the embryo until the placenta is formed. The amnion will grow into the amniotic sac and fill with fluid to protect the baby.

In the meantime, the embryo's cells are setting up to perform specialized jobs. Some cells will become bones, muscles, and internal organs, while others will form the circulatory or nervous

DID YOU KNOW?

Prenatal yoga is wonderful for you and your pregnant partner. Yoga increases circulation, which increases blood flow and provides oxygen to mom and baby. Yoga also promotes relaxation and increases concentration, which help control anxiety related to being pregnant. Flexibility and balance—which can become a problem as mom's center of gravity shifts throughout your pregnancy—will improve as well. Finally, prenatal yoga can help ease backaches, combat insomnia, and help you and mom relax.

✚ HEALTH CONCERNS

If you or your partner are smokers, now is the time to quit. Smoking is associated with at least 115,000 miscarriages each year in the U.S. Additionally, smoking causes low birth weight and can stunt growth in utero. Exposure to secondhand smoke in utero makes infants more prone to respiratory illnesses and more likely to succumb to Sudden Infant Death Syndrome (SIDS). With a new baby on the way, there is no better time to quit for good. Visit www.smokefree.gov to get helpful tips and advice.

systems. Around the third lunar week the embryo flattens into a disc that has a dark line called the primitive streak. This is where the cells that make up baby's brain and spinal cord will eventually develop. Other cells are developing into 3 layers called the endoderm, ectoderm, and mesoderm. Each of these plays an important role in baby's development. The outer layer is the ectoderm and is responsible for producing the neural tube from which the spine and brain will develop. The inner layer, or endoderm, is where the lungs, intestines, and bladder will grow. The middle layer, the mesoderm, is where baby's heart and circulatory system are already forming. Indeed, your baby is in the most crucial period of heart development. Heart folds fuse together to form a tube that, by month's end, develops into a 4-chambered pump that starts to beat.

WHAT TO EXPECT
DR.S VISITS

The only test to expect this month is an at-home pregnancy test and perhaps a urine or blood test at the doctor's office to confirm the results.

What's Happening: Dad

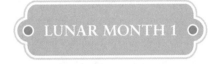

First Trimester

A MAN'S REACTION TO THE NEWS that he is going to be a father may range from elation to panic and include every emotion in between. No matter what your first response is, you can expect to experience a range of emotions in these first few weeks as you adjust to the news. The following sections will help you to get a handle on what to expect as both you and your partner adjust to your new status as parents-to-be.

WHAT DAD IS THINKING AND FEELING

What is dad thinking and feeling? In a word: everything. Finding out you are going to be a father causes you to experience emotions you didn't know were possible. Pregnancy may raise questions about your role as partner, provider, father, and son. You may also begin to ponder concerns such as global warming. When all of these issues surface at once, they give rise to uncomfortable—and constantly changing—feelings about your identity, your relationship with your father, and the state of the world. This rollercoaster of emotions is due, in part, to your changing priorities and the very short time in which you have to adjust to them.

One reason for flighty emotions is that pregnancy is a confusing time for men who do not usually analyze their relationships with people. Becoming a father lends itself to looking back over your own childhood and thinking about the kind of man your father was. This can inform many of the choices you make as a parent. Some dads-to-be base their parenting style heavily on their own fathers, while others make decisions in opposition to how they were raised. The majority of men, though, choose the best of their father's parenting and leave the rest in the past.

Working through issues you had with your father might make you feel anxious about what kind of dad you will become. In fact, it is common to oscillate between feeling completely incompetent and envisioning yourself as "father of the year." This kind of insecurity is normal for first-time dads, and does not mean you are destined to ruin your child's life. On the contrary, such thoughtfulness indicates a genuine interest in the exploration of your role as father and the kind of man you want to be for your child.

As you consider the kind of man you are and want to become, it is natural to wonder how your relationship with your partner will change. As with other pregnancy-related issues, feelings about your relationship will morph into something else by the time baby is born. Therefore, it is normal to feel a renewed adoration for your partner upon discovering she is pregnant—or to feel slightly intimidated by her immediate connection to the pregnancy. You may look at her, knowing she is carrying your child, and feel a great need to protect her. This may result in a lack of sexual attraction or the desire for constant affection. You may feel all of these things at once, or they may come and go throughout the pregnancy. Just remember, however you feel about your partner this month will likely be very different in the months to follow.

Interestingly, your feelings about safety and world events will likely change over the course of the pregnancy. For example, many fathers

✖ FOOD FOR THOUGHT

Help your partner start her pregnancy out right by having healthy and nutritious snacks in the house. Figs make wonderful snacks, are healthy, and can help her fight the discomfort of first-trimester constipation. If it is not too hard on her stomach, orange juice is a great addition to her mid-morning snack, because it includes vitamin C and is often fortified with calcium. Yogurt is another healthy and easy snack that will give mom a mid-afternoon energy boost, since it has protein and is also a great source of calcium.

find they now care more about how many airbags a car has rather than how fast it accelerates onto the freeway. And for fathers-to-be, issues in the news regarding crime, politics, the environment, economics, war, and medical insurance often supercede sports scores and first-round draft picks. Indeed, becoming a father can be a wake-up call for a man who wants his child to inherit all of the best parts of society, and none of the worst. If this shift in consciousness causes you anxiety, you are not alone, and it does not mean you are weak. All it means is that you are a human being who is about to become a parent!

THINGS DAD SHOULD KNOW

The first month of pregnancy is strange for dad. He knows his partner is pregnant, but there may not be physical evidence of that yet if she has no symptoms. Therefore, life still seems pretty much the same, though change is definitely in the air. And since there is nothing physical to connect with yet this month, dad must find other ways to feel included.

DID YOU KNOW?

There are several tricks you can use to help mom deal with nausea. For instance, carry around a few lemon slices or lemon-flavored candies in your pocket. This way, if she is exposed to odors that cause her to feel sick, she can inhale the scent of lemon instead. This has been shown to prevent the escalation of nausea to vomiting. You should also carry around black licorice for her to nibble on when her stomach is giving her trouble. Sipping peppermint tea also helps, as will inhaling peppermint oil.

Thus, you can get plugged in to the pregnancy zone by understanding the following bits of information:

- At-home pregnancy tests measure hCG levels after the fertilized egg implants itself in the uterus. Therefore, if your partner tests too soon, the results may be negative. For accuracy, she should wait until she misses her next period— about 6 to 12 days after fertilization.

- Three out of four miscarriages occur within the first 10 days of fertilization due to failed implantation, which results in menstruation. Many couples never even know they were pregnant.

- Doctors calculate your partner's due date based on her last menstrual period (LMP) but she is not actually pregnant until implantation occurs. As a result, pregnancy based on LMP calculations lasts 40 weeks, whereas lunar, or actual gestation, is 38 weeks.

- On average, pregnancy lasts about 266 days, but healthcare providers measure gestation in weeks.

- Though your partner may not experience any symptoms yet, hormones are hard at work causing changes to her breasts, uterus, and cervix.
- Fluctuating hormone levels can cause your partner to experience extreme mood swings.
- Your partner's heart is beginning to pump more blood to supply nutrients and oxygen to the embryo.
- By the end of the first month, the embryo has already started to develop the earliest versions of its major internal organs.
- Your partner will probably gain between 25 and 35 pounds over the course of the pregnancy.

As each month slips by, new information will build upon what you learned in the previous month. There may be months when nothing much happens—such as early in the third trimester—and months where it seems as though your wife and baby are growing larger by the minute. Just try to take it all in stride and do your best to keep up!

HELPFUL HINTS FOR DAD

Some men feel like they are unable to keep up with all of the information and body changes their partners go through during pregnancy. But in order to feel connected to your partner and the pregnancy, you must pay close attention before you get too far behind.

This list will help you to get oriented and dig in.
- Get involved in the pregnancy from the beginning
- Offer to buy the pregnancy test
- Be there when your partner uses it
- Help choose a healthcare provider
- Go to as many prenatal appointments as possible

✖ TIPS & ADVICE

If you've been trying to get pregnant for awhile, mom has probably already started taking prenatal vitamins. However, if she hasn't, now is the time to start. Folate is necessary for rapid cell production and can be ingested by eating leafy, green vegetables like spinach, beans, and peas. It is also found in fortified breakfast cereals. However, most women are unable to eat enough of these foods to get the right amount of folate, so it is necessary to get the recommended daily dose (400 micrograms) in supplement form.

- Educate yourself about pregnancy, labor, and childbirth
- Find out how much coverage your insurance company offers during pregnancy
- Get familiar with pregnancy vocabulary
- Investigate your options for taking time off once baby is born
- Listen to your partner
- Share your thoughts and feelings
- Provide her with the food and drink she craves
- Get advice from other dads
- Seek advice from sisters or friends who have children
- Avoid taking on additional responsibilities at work
- Exercise daily—with your partner if possible
- Get enough rest
- Eat healthy meals
- Quit smoking
- Reduce alcohol consumption
- Remind your partner to take her prenatal vitamins
- Avoid sharing morbid pregnancy stories with your partner
- Be considerate of your partner's needs when making social or

travel plans
- Practice relaxation exercises
- Remember to hug and kiss your partner

Many of these tips may not come naturally to every father-to-be, so refer back to them when you feel at a loss for action or words. When in doubt, pick up this book and start reading!

COMMON QUESTIONS THAT DADS HAVE

In the first month of pregnancy your questions will be very different from those that surface during the last month. At this stage, you are likely concerned with issues such as your readiness to be a parent, fear of miscarriage, and what will happen to the dynamic between you and your partner.

The most common questions at this stage include:
Am I ready to be a father? It is impossible to say whether any man is ever ready to be a father. No man (or woman) is born with the knowledge it takes to raise a child. It must be learned over time. Rest assured that at some point your instincts will kick in and you will be able to intuit most of your baby's needs. Also, you learn from your parents, family members, friends, and books. You observe, pick and choose what suits you, and then do your best. Think of being a parent as an ever-evolving job that takes a lifetime of trial and error, risk, and reward.

What if my partner has a miscarriage? About 20 percent of pregnancies end in miscarriage during the first 20 weeks of gestation. Some believe the statistic is as high as 50 percent when you factor in the failed implantations that occur within the first 10 days (which mom may never know about). However, if you already know your partner is pregnant, the latter statistic does not

---

ⓘ PREGNANCY FACT

Alcohol and drug consumption can interfere with the implantation process and cause a miscarriage. In fact, researchers estimate that between 7 and 10 days after conception is when the embryo is at the highest risk for failed implantation. Therefore, you and mom should stop drinking before becoming pregnant. Later in the pregnancy, you can discuss with your doctor whether it is OK for mom to have a glass of wine now and then, but it is crucial that she abstain during this critical stage of development.

---

apply. Therefore there is an 80 percent chance your partner will not miscarry. There is no doubt the first trimester is a nail-biting time for expectant couples. Measures your partner can take to reduce her risk of miscarriage include quitting smoking, limiting caffeine intake, avoiding alcohol consumption, steering clear of secondhand smoke, avoiding certain medications, and getting good prenatal care.

How will our relationship change during pregnancy?
How much your relationship changes during pregnancy is due, in large part, to how well you communicate with each other. For example, if you feel disconnected from your partner but do not tell her, the distance will continue to grow. However, if you discuss the pregnancy's impact on your relationship it can be cathartic and reaffirming for both partners.

What if I am not attracted to my partner? The chances of this happening are slim. The majority of men find their pregnant partner extremely sexy and voluptuous while carrying their child — even when the mother-to-be feels as big as a house. A few men will be turned off by their partner's weight gain, but that won't happen for a while. At this stage, your partner looks the same as she usually does. If you are turned off by the idea that your baby is growing inside of her, this may be a bit more challenging to overcome. Try to block out the images that bother you, and see your partner as the woman you love, who is helping build your family. If you're having a hard time with mom's new look and size, shower her with compliments and give yourself time to adjust. Never hurt her feelings by saying you're not as attracted to her as you once were! She is very sensitive and feeling overwhelmed already. Spend quality time with her and remember that she will get back to her pre-pregnancy size soon enough.

HOW DAD CAN DEAL

Finding out you are going to be a dad may feel something like being in the middle of a tornado. And as your life seems to spin out of control, you'll need to get anchored and centered.

✚ HEALTH CONCERNS

Although experts generally agree that the amount of caffeine in a 8-ounce cup of coffee is not harmful, caffeine in larger amounts may cause miscarriages or result in low-birth weight babies. In some cases, babies born to women who consumed more than 500 mg of caffeine per day had breathing problems and faster heartbeats than those born to women who consumed less or abstained all together. Thus, experts make a general recommendation that mom should limit her caffeine intake to 300 mg or less per day.

Here are some suggestions for how to deal with life during the first month of pregnancy:

- Exercise on your lunch break. Exercise is an excellent way to reduce stress, increase health, and burn off nervous energy. Besides, starting now sets the tone for leading a healthier lifestyle throughout pregnancy and after your child is born.

- Eat a healthy snack every few hours. One moody partner is enough for most households, so avoid the late-afternoon sugar crash by eating small, frequent meals and avoiding excessive amounts of caffeine and sugar.

- Go to bed earlier. You have many sleepless nights in your future, so catch your zzz's while you can. Studies show adults need at least 7 or 8 hours of sleep for their bodies and minds to heal and recharge.

- Take 20 minutes to decompress before you walk in the door. Once you walk into the house your partner is likely to be in full baby-planning mode. Before you go home, take a quick walk, drive around, run an errand, or have a cup of coffee. Doing so will reduce the risk of snappy miscommunications when you get home.

- Remember to breathe. When feeling stressed, people often take shallow breaths that actually increase heart rate and exacerbate agitation. So breathe deeply and often. Count to 5 on each inhale and exhale several times a day.

- Stretch. Stretching releases tension and reminds you to connect with your physical status. For example, if you work in front of a computer, stretch on the hour. Doing so will ward off stiff muscles and headaches.

- Talk to a friend. Between work and planning for a baby, your life is probably pretty busy. But don't let your friends drift away. Men need companionship, and getting together a couple of times a month is often just what is needed.

One change during pregnancy is the temporary worsening of your partner's vision. Pregnancy-related blurred vision is caused by a temporary thickening of the cornea as well as by a decrease in fluid pressure in the eyes. Other eye-related symptoms include dry eyes and puffy lids. These symptoms are usually normal and will disappear after birth. However, a sudden change in mom's vision can be a sign of a serious problem, such as diabetes or hypertension, and should be shared with your doctor immediately.

Above all, take time to yourself while you still can. Though your partner will need you to do more around the house as the pregnancy progresses, you should still carve out 30 minutes each day that is just for you. Use that time to listen to music, exercise, play guitar, work in the garage, read, catch up with a friend, or just veg on the couch for a while. Claiming this time each day will help you stay calm in crises and benefit your overall health and disposition.

HOW DAD CAN HELP

The first month of pregnancy is a critical time for your baby's heart and circulatory system development. It makes sense, therefore, that your partner should eat a healthy diet, rich in nutrients and vitamins. However, this may not be possible once pregnancy sickness really kicks in. So, now is the time to help enrich your partner's diet by stepping up as shopper and chef. This role does not come naturally to many men, but it is one that will be extremely helpful to your partner.

Your first task is to learn what nutrients are essential for this early stage of development—and then to prepare tasty meals out of nutritious ingredients. It really is not as hard as it sounds, and if you plan ahead and shop right you will figure out a couple staple meals that taste good, too.

The following list of vitamins, essential nutrients, and the foods that contain them will help get you started:

Calcium: The FDA recommends pregnant women consume 1,000 milligrams of calcium each day. Calcium helps baby form strong bones, teeth, and healthy organs, like the heart. Calcium also gets baby to establish a normal heart rhythm and to perform healthy blood clotting. Calcium-rich foods include low-fat dairy products, tofu, calcium-fortified orange juice, cereals, and whole grain breads.

Iron: The Centers for Disease Control recommends that pregnant women consume 27 milligrams of iron daily. Iron is essential to hemoglobin production, which carries oxygen in the blood throughout the body and will keep mom from becoming anemic. Iron-rich foods include red meat, beans, pumpkin seeds, potatoes with skin, and fortified cereals.

Folic Acid: The American Pregnancy Association recommends pregnant women consume 400 micrograms of folic acid a day. Studies show a decrease in neurological birth defects when mom gets the daily recommended dose early in the first trimester. Since it is nearly impossible to get this amount from food, remind your partner to take a prenatal vitamin daily. Foods rich in folic acid include liver, egg yolks, legumes, lentils, almonds, sweet potatoes, spinach, Brussels sprouts, bananas, oranges, and peaches.

Protein: The FDA recommends pregnant women consume 60 grams of protein each day. You can easily provide the recommended

Mom's blood volume will increase by up to 50 percent by the time she is ready to deliver baby. Thus, it is recommended that she increase her water intake to stay hydrated, since her heart works 40 percent harder than before she was pregnant. In some cases, the extra weight means that sleeping on her back can put pressure on an artery that can slow or stop blood flow to the lower half of your body. Therefore, it is also recommended that mom sleep on her left side to ensure maximum blood flow to the uterus.

daily dose by making dishes that feature lean meats, eggs, lentils, dried beans, cheese, nuts, or tofu.

Omega-3s: The Omega-3 polyunsaturated fatty acid DHA (docosahexaenoic acid) is necessary for eye development and brain growth. Including oily fish in your partner's diet, such as wild salmon and sardines, DHA-rich eggs, walnuts, and flaxseeds, will provide this essential nutrient.

Fat: Fat is necessary for your partner's diet, so avoid fat-free products. Plus, some vitamins (A, D, E, and K) are fat-soluble, which means they require a certain amount of fat to be absorbed by the body. Focus on monounsaturated and polyunsaturated fats—the "good fats" found in salmon, trout, herring, avocados, olives, walnuts, and oils such as soybean, corn, safflower, canola, olive, and sunflower.

Use this information as your starting point to make a shopping list that includes a variety of protein sources as well as fresh fruits and vegetables. Keep in mind that it is inadvisable to make large batches of any meal since your partner's taste tolerance may change from day to day. However, always purchase healthy snacks, such as carrot and celery sticks, yogurt, almonds, string cheese, and fruit so your partner never has to scramble when she is feeling hungry.

HOW DAD CAN BE INVOLVED

The best way to be involved in the pregnancy is to ask your partner what she needs. At this early stage, however, she may have no idea what that might be. So, stand by and wait for instructions.

Here are a few things you can do to get connected:

- Join an online dads' group
- Rub or kiss your partner's belly every morning and night
- Research big-ticket baby gear, such as car seats, strollers, and cribs
- Eat a pregnancy diet with your partner
- Give up the same vices she is giving up
- Go with your partner to interview potential healthcare providers—and have questions ready to go

The thing with pregnancy is that you can be as involved as you want to be, so if you want to know something, find out. If you want to touch your partner's belly, tell her. If you wonder what it feels like to be pregnant, ask her to explain it to you. There is no rule in the Book of How to Be a Man that states men must be silent and sidelined during pregnancy. After all, you are living in an age when the majority of couples say "We're pregnant," so there is no excuse for you not to be involved if you want to be.

DAD'S RESPONSIBILITIES

Your primary responsibility in the first month of pregnancy is to

ⓘ PREGNANCY FACT

Iron is critical for mom, because it is required for hemoglobin production, which carries oxygen in the blood throughout the body. In order to avoid mom becoming anemic during her second or third trimesters, the Centers for Disease Control recommends that pregnant women consume 27 milligrams of iron. Cook mom meals with iron-rich foods, such as red meat, beans, pumpkin seeds, potatoes with skin, and fortified cereals. It is also very important to make sure she is taking her prenatal vitamins daily.

adjust to the news that you are going to be a father. This may be a quick process if you were trying for a baby or a slow one if the pregnancy was a surprise.

One way to digest the idea is to use positive visualizations:

- Imagine rocking your baby to sleep
- Picture your wife nursing your baby in the first light of morning
- Hear yourself announcing your child's name to family and friends
- Imagine looking at her 10 tiny fingers and toes for the first time
- Picture reading a story to your son or daughter
- Imagine your child's first birthday party
- See yourself teaching your child to play piano
- Envision your child scoring a goal at soccer practice
- Feel the pride of watching your child go through graduation

✖ TIPS & ADVICE

Consult your doctor before your partner takes any medications—this includes over-the-counter drugs like acetaminophen, ibuprofen, and cold medicines. If she gets a cold or the flu, most remedies will unfortunately be off limits. The FDA breaks down drug safety into letter-based categories from A to X. A is the safest, while X indicates that a pregnant woman should not take the medicine under any circumstances. When filling a prescription, always ask which letter the medication falls under.

This exercise has hopefully helped you feel more comfortable with adding "father" to the list of roles you already play in your life. With time, you'll be as good at being a father as you are at everything else.

Lunar Month

Two

First Trimester

Lunar Month two . . . .

MONTHLY TO-DO LISTS

☐ Attend the first prenatal meeting with mom

☐ Have a list of questions ready to ask the doctor

☐ Note that mom's increasing morning sickness may last all day

☐ Take on duties mom is too sick to handle, like cooking and cleaning

☐ Take over administering any medication to other kids or animals that could seep through mom's skin and endanger the baby

☐ Spend extra time with your other children

☐ Expect your partner to be very moody

☐ Help mom get essential nutrients by preparing healthy meals

☐ Establish a baby budget

MY PERSONAL CHECKLIST:

☐ ....

☐ ....

☐ ....

MY HOPES FOR THIS MONTH:

....

....

....

....

....

....

....

....

....

....

....

What's Happening: Mom & Baby

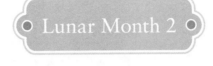

○ Lunar Month 2 ○

First Trimester

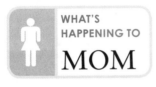

WHAT'S HAPPENING TO MOM

By the end of this month, your partner will definitely "feel" pregnant. She will likely suffer from some persistent and nasty symptoms, and may gain a little weight. These physical signs of pregnancy will help her settle into the pregnancy mentally. This reality check may send her into emotional overdrive—and you with her. But before you run for cover, consider extending a little more empathy than you're used to. The symptoms that hammer more than 70 percent of pregnant women in the second month can be relentless and hard to manage.

One early and fairly constant symptom during pregnancy is intense heartburn. Heartburn affects more than 25 percent of pregnant women and is caused by stomach acids that rise up into the esophagus, which relaxes during pregnancy. As a result, your partner may have a constant burning sensation from her stomach up into her throat. She can minimize this discomfort by eating several small meals a day. Sitting up for at least an hour after eating can help too. Also this month, mom's stomach will be increasingly hemmed in by her growing uterus. To compensate for the crowding, her midsection will thicken just enough to make her waistband feel uncomfortable. Though she is not ready to wear maternity

MOM'S
Symptoms

- Nausea and vomiting
- Fatigue
- Dizziness
- Frequent urination
- Constipation
- Gas
- Bloating
- Heartburn
- Indigestion
- Aversions to certain foods and smells
- Cravings
- Breast sensitivity
- Vaginal discharge
- Headaches
- Mood swings

clothes, encourage her to wear soft, stretchy waistbands because tight clothing can exacerbate heartburn.

Wearing loose-fitting clothing will help your partner with another embarrassing problem this month: gas. By the end of mom's eighth week of pregnancy, her uterus has doubled in size and her system is circulating extra fluid. This causes pressure to mount on her intestines, making her feel bloated and gassy. In addition to being embarrassing, these conditions are painful. She may need to pass gas frequently in order to feel relief. Most women eventually get used to passing gas, but before you start cracking jokes, check in with your partner's mood—she may not think farting is as funny as you do!

In addition to heartburn and gas, your partner is likely to experience some level of nausea this month—usually around the sixth week. It may be confined to the minutes after she first wakes up, or last all day long. She may have low-grade queasiness or feel the need to vomit every time she eats or drinks. Intermittent nausea is exhausting and unpleasant, but completely normal. What is not normal, however, is if your partner throws up continuously or loses weight very quickly. In this case, she may be among the 1 percent of pregnant women who suffer from hyperemesis gravidarum, or severe pregnancy sickness. This condition requires immediate medical attention.

This month heralds other symptoms that may increase your partner's nausea: the development of a heightened sense of smell, headaches, hot flashes, and dizziness. Most of these symptoms occur as a result of estrogen flooding her system and will remain with her throughout the pregnancy. Therefore, your once-alluring cologne may have to sit on the shelf until baby is born to prevent your partner from puking when you enter the room.

Additionally, your partner's sex drive may take a nosedive this month. Besides not feeling well, her breasts are probably sensitive, and she may have a thick, white vaginal discharge. Called leukorrhea, this discharge is caused by increased levels of estrogen and blood flow to the vaginal area. It is a normal pregnancy symptom, but it can be unpleasant and make your partner self-conscious about having intercourse. However, if your partner is in the mood for sex,

ⓘ PREGNANCY FACT

Back pain is a very common ailment for pregnant women. There are many causes—weight gain, hormonal surges, and a shifting center of gravity. To help ease your partner's back pain, purchase a body pillow for her to sleep with between her knees while lying on her left side. You can also help by exercising with her at whatever level your doctor has approved. Taking action early in the pregnancy can help to mediate extreme lower back pain during and after labor.

it is safe. By now, a mucus plug has formed that seals mom's cervix and protects baby from infection. Go easy if you do make love, because the cervix, swollen from the excess fluid in her body, can be sensitive to touch and even prone to bleeding. Therefore, when it comes to sex, let your partner be your guide.

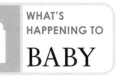

WHAT'S HAPPENING TO BABY

Over the course of the next month your baby will undergo great changes that will make him look less like a tadpole and more like a tiny human. Development is kicked into high gear as mom's body produces another important hormone called human placental lactogen (HPL). HPL originates from the placenta. It acts as a growth hormone for baby and breaks down sugars and proteins in the maternal blood so that he can digest them. As the nutrition transfer system gets up and running, baby starts to grow at an astonishing speed.

This month your baby graduates from the embryonic stage into the fetal stage of development. There is a lot more to this process than just a change in terminology. For example, he starts to form the early stages of his facial features, including his otic (ear) and nasal pits. His eyes take shape, though their final color will not be set until a week or so after birth. Also, as baby's arms and legs form, one of your baby's most curious embryonic features will disappear: his tail! If you didn't already know, all human embryos have a tail. As they grow, the tail is absorbed by the rest of the body—and that is what is happening to your little one this month. The absence of his tail adds to his human appearance. Moreover, by month's end, baby will already have his one-of-a-kind fingerprints. And though your partner will not yet feel it, his fingers, toes, arms and legs will soon flutter around in the amniotic fluid.

One out of every 200 pregnant women will develop a condition called hyperemesis gravidarum—severe nausea and vomiting. This is different from normal pregnancy sickness in that morning sickness usually eases up around the 14th week. Hyperemesis gravidarum, however, often lasts throughout the pregnancy and causes such severe nausea and vomiting that mom is unable to consume enough calories and nutrients. Your doctor can provide treatment for this condition should your partner suffer from it.

In addition to external features, exciting changes are happening internally, too. All of baby's internal organs will have their basic form by the end of the month, with some even beginning to function. Though his lungs will not be mature until late in the third trimester, they will resemble a tiny set of adult lungs in just a few weeks. And by the end of the month, baby's heartbeat will be so strong it can be seen and heard on an ultrasound.

**WHAT TO EXPECT
DR.S VISITS**

Your first prenatal appointment will be scheduled around 8 to 10 weeks after your partner's last period. At this appointment, your partner will get a physical exam. She will also provide a urine sample so the doctor can see if there is an elevated presence of ketones, sugar, or protein, which may require further testing to rule out gestational diabetes or kidney problems. Urine tests also indicate whether any infections are brewing.

Mom will also undergo an internal exam. The doctor will insert a speculum into her vagina followed by a cotton swab—this is called a pap smear and checks for precancerous cells on the cervix. Another specimen is taken to test for STDs. She will also visually and manually check your partner's cervix and the size of her uterus to determine how far along she is. The doctor will insert 2 fingers into your partner's vagina to measure her birth canal and check for any abnormalities, such as a tilted uterus.

Blood is drawn at this visit to determine your partner's blood type and rhesus factor, which is either Rh positive or Rh negative. If your partner is Rh negative she will be given a Rh immunoglobulin shot once during pregnancy and once after delivery. The doctor will also check mom's white and red blood cell counts and check for German measles/rubella immunity and hepatitis B. Other blood screenings may be performed to test for HIV, syphilis, cystic fibrosis, sickle-cell disease, Tay-Sachs, and thalassemia. In some cases, dad may also be asked to submit to a blood test if the risk for any of the above conditions is high.

At this visit you will also get to hear your baby's heartbeat for the first time, thanks to a Doppler, or heart monitor. The device looks like a microphone that the doctor moves around your partner's belly until the baby's heartbeat is detected. Prepare to be amazed! For many parents, this is the first moment of true connection to the baby.

What's Happening: Dad

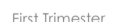

Lunar Month 2

First Trimester

In many ways, the second month is much the same for you, since mom does not really look pregnant. This makes having a baby still more of a concept for dads than a reality. You may also find yourself afraid to get attached to the idea of having a baby in case a problem develops with the pregnancy. This is normal for many men at this point.

WHAT DAD IS THINKING AND FEELING

In the second month of pregnancy, dad's mind starts to wander toward who this creature growing in his partner's womb might become. He ponders baby's gender and possible future, imagining holidays, birthdays, recitals, graduations, and the friends and partners his child may have. In short, he begins to think about all of the potential he helped to create. But he may also be filled with terror that his wife will miscarry, that a disease or deformity will befall his child, or that his partner will die during childbirth. These are all common thoughts that will likely accompany you throughout the pregnancy.

However, the first thought that usually blips across the screen is, "Do I want a boy or girl?" This is a common question and one that people over the past six decades have answered similarly. In

As a general rule, a pregnant woman should avoid any activity that raises her body temperature to 102 degrees or more. Studies have shown that it is particularly dangerous to the developing embryo or fetus in the early stages of pregnancy. Thus, mom should avoid exercising during the hottest part of the day. Also, she should avoid hot tubs and saunas, both of which can make her prone to dizzy spells, fainting, and dehydration. Pregnant women are already at risk for experiencing these symptoms, and don't need more of them.

1941, the Gallup organization polled expectant American couples to learn whether they preferred to have a son or daughter. Back then, 38 percent of respondents wanted a son, 24 percent wanted a daughter, and 38 percent had no preference. In 2003, Gallup conducted the same poll and learned the results had not changed much. Regardless of what you end up with, chances are that you, like those polled by Gallup, have given at least some thought to whether you would prefer a son or daughter.

It is common for a man to imagine himself in various scenarios with his little girl or boy. This is particularly tempting for men who had an especially happy or disappointing childhood. In fact, many parents view having a child as an opportunity to right the wrongs of their past or to propagate the parts of childhood they appreciated. This response to pregnancy is normal and usually targeted toward a particular gender. For example, if you had an absentee father, you may long for a son with whom you can do the fatherly things you missed out on. While there is nothing inherently wrong with fantasizing about football tosses with your son, getting too attached to having a boy can make finding out a daughter is on the way fall on disappointed ears.

And though you are a few months away from being able to learn the gender of your child, it can be difficult to control your feelings about your preferences. You may even feel guilty knowing you have always wanted a daughter and, thus, fear the disappointment of having a son. Still, other men truly have no preference and hope only for a healthy child and a safe delivery for their partner.

THINGS DAD SHOULD KNOW

After the first prenatal appointment you may feel like pregnancy requires you to speak a foreign language. There are many new concepts and terms that most men find bewildering at first. By next month, however, you will be measuring time in weeks and speaking like you've been expecting a baby for years.

Here are some pregnancy concepts and terms to get you started:

Amniotic fluid: Water and other liquid that surrounds the fetus

Amniotic sac: The membrane that houses the amniotic fluid, fetus, and placenta

Ectopic pregnancy: When fertilization occurs outside of the uterus, such as in the fallopian tubes

Embryonic period: The first 10 weeks of baby's development

Endometrium: Thickened uterine wall in which the baby first burrows during implantation

DID YOU KNOW?

Ultrasounds are a safe, noninvasive way to monitor your baby's progress in utero. An ultrasound creates a picture by using high-frequency sound waves. Echoes are transformed into black-and-white images that are viewed on a monitor. The test is performed as needed throughout pregnancy by your doctor. A topical wand will be used on the outside of your partner's belly or inserted into the vagina. This can also offer more information if your doctor suspects a problem or wants to confirm the due date.

Fetal anomaly: Abnormal development of a fetus

Gestation: The time between conception and birth of a child, lasting approximately 266 days, or 38 weeks

Neural tube defects: Abnormal development of the spine and brain that occurs during early stages of fetal growth

Ossification: Bone growth

Perinatologist: A doctor who specializes in high-risk pregnancies

Pica: When mom has the desire to chew or eat nonfood items, such as clay, dirt, or pennies. This is not healthy and should be reported to your partner's healthcare provider.

Placenta: An organ created by mom's body during pregnancy. Nutrients are provided by the placenta while toxins are filtered out. Some toxins, such as alcohol, can get to baby even after being filtered through the placenta.

Round ligament pain: Abdominal pain associated with the stretching of the uterus during pregnancy

Spontaneous abortion: Pregnancy is naturally terminated by mom's body within the first 20 weeks

Stretch marks: Long, red lines that may appear on a woman's stomach, hips, breasts, and thighs as her skin stretches during pregnancy

Teratogens: Harmful substances, such as alcohol and drugs that can damage a developing fetus

Trimesters: The three measurements into which pregnancy is broken down. Each trimester is made up of 3 months, and each month has 4 weeks. The first trimester is months 1 to 3, the second is 4 to 6, the third is 7 to 9 (or longer if the pregnancy goes past the due date).

These terms should get you through until next month when other terms come to the forefront. Feel free to memorize the terms you don't know and dazzle your partner with your pregnancy knowledge!

HELPFUL HINTS FOR DAD

One of the best ways to support your partner this month and in the months that follow is to understand the dos and don'ts of the

Your pregnant partner should completely avoid most herbal products. Certain herbs, such as St. John's wort and black cohosh, can stimulate uterine contractions and cause a miscarriage. Essential oils made from herbs can also be dangerous. These include rosemary, cinnamon, fennel, oregano, and sage. Since the Food and Drug Administration does not regulate herbal remedies, one can never be sure what is in an herbal product. Play it safe and be sure mom avoids all herbal products.

pregnancy diet. Once you have a handle on foods that support pregnancy, try to eat as she does—within reason, of course.

Here are some helpful hints for dining as your partner should:

- Do eat a variety of fresh fruits and vegetables
- Do eat 4 to 5 servings of dairy products daily
- Do eat 2 to 4 servings of fruit
- Do eat 6 to 11 servings of complex carbohydrates
- Do eat a high fiber diet
- Do make a meal plan with your partner
- Do cook poultry and other meats thoroughly to avoid salmonella
- Do eat several small meals each day
- Do have healthy snacks ready to go
- Do entertain your partner's cravings
- Do respect her aversions
- Do encourage your partner to drink 8 to 10 glasses of water a day

- Do use ginger, lemon, and peppermint in the kitchen to help ease nausea
- Don't buy foods that contain artificial sweeteners
- Don't offer to pick up fast food more than once a week
- Don't eat for two
- Don't eat more than 3 to 5 servings of fat in a day
- Don't eat fish with high mercury content, such as tuna, shark, and swordfish
- Don't eat sushi or raw shellfish
- Don't stock the kitchen with junk food
- Don't eat unpasteurized dairy products, such as brie, Camembert, and feta as they may contain the harmful bacteria listeriosis

Following these basic guidelines in the kitchen for the next several months will make your partner feel less alone in her food choices and allow you to participate in the health of your baby's development. Indeed, sharing meals is definitely an area in which couples can be a team during pregnancy.

ⓘ PREGNANCY FACT

If you have a cat, you should assume kitty litter duty for the rest of the pregnancy. In fact, mom should have limited contact with the cat until her pregnancy is over, because cat feces can carry the dangerous toxoplasmosis virus. Keep in mind that indoor cats who use litter boxes can track the virus all over the house, so it is important that you keep the house extremely clean by vacuuming and mopping constantly. Consider moving the litter box to a part of the house mom rarely visits, such as the basement or boiler room.

✖ FOOD FOR THOUGHT

Pregnancy is a great time to go organic. Commercially grown foods contain harmful pesticides that can cross the placenta and enter your baby's bloodstream. In fact, research has linked these chemicals to cancer and other diseases. Organic products can be quite expensive, so if you have to prioritize, make the following items organic: milk, meat, nectarines, pears, peaches, apples, cherries, strawberries, imported grapes, spinach, potatoes, bell peppers, and raspberries.

COMMON QUESTIONS THAT DADS HAVE

Most men go to the doctor so infrequently that the idea of monthly checkups might seem excessive. But prenatal care is an important way to ensure that both your partner and baby are healthy. It can be common for dads to feel invisible at these checkups. However, showing up prepared with a list of questions for the doctor will establish you as an interested father and a person to be taken seriously. In addition, developing rapport with the staff by remembering names and faces makes them more inclined to return your phone calls and pay attention to you at the appointments.

Some common questions dads have about prenatal checkups include:

How often do I have to go to these appointments? If the pregnancy is progressing normally, your partner will see her doctor once a month until the last half of the third trimester. At that point, the doctor usually sees mom every two weeks, then once a week until labor starts. You should attend as many of these appointments as possible. Doing so deepens your connection to the pregnancy, shows your partner that you support her, and also presents a united front to the doctor and staff. If work is an issue, ask mom to schedule an appointment during your lunch hour so you can come for at least part of it. It is also perfectly acceptable to miss one now and then.

How long are the appointments? Allot between 2 and 3 hours for the first prenatal checkup. Each appointment thereafter should last 30 minutes or less, depending on whether the doctor is on schedule and how many questions you ask.

Why is the first appointment so long? The first prenatal appointment takes a long time because there is a lot to cover. The doctor will do a physical exam on your partner in addition to blood and urine tests. Moreover, if you have requested it, there may be a genetic counseling evaluation to determine the risks of certain hereditary diseases. This is also the time when parents have the most questions, so doctors set aside more time to answer them. Take full advantage of this appointment, because those that follow will fly by.

What if I don't like my partner's doctor? What's more important is whether your partner likes her doctor. It will be annoying if you and the doctor do not get along, but it will be disastrous if your partner has issues with him. Chances are, if the doctor rubs you the wrong way, your partner feels the same. Talk to her about it and remind her it is not too late to change physicians and find someone with whom you both feel comfortable.

Do I have to report sexually transmitted diseases (STDs) to my partner's doctor? Yes. Though it will be uncomfortable, even humiliating, you must report any STDs since those carried by you have likely been contracted by your partner. Letting the doctor know about them is necessary to both your partner and baby's health. For example, if you gave your partner herpes, developing vaginal sores can infect the baby during delivery, making a Cesarean a better, safer option.

What if I don't know my family medical history? There are many reasons for not knowing your family medical history, such as being adopted or having estranged or deceased parents. Though it is helpful in predicting potential problems, it is not necessary to have this information. And, over the course of the pregnancy, your partner will be offered many tests that can determine whether your child is at risk for certain hereditary diseases.

Is it appropriate to ask the doctor about sex during pregnancy? Yes! Definitely ask the doctor any and all questions you have regarding the health and safety of your partner and baby. However embarrassed you may feel in the moment should not stop you from having confidence to engage in a healthy sex life with your partner over the next several months.

HOW DAD CAN DEAL

Some time after the first prenatal appointment, dad may start to notice mom digging into her pregnancy. She may be distracted and focus only on what goes in her body and what she must avoid. This is normal behavior brought on by the tremendous responsibility mom feels to protect and enhance her baby's development. Her intent concentration may have you feeling left out in the cold. One way to deal with this chill factor is to warm things up between you and your partner. Indeed, mom can become so consumed by her pregnancy that she forgets to hug, kiss, or touch you for days—even weeks. Know that it is not personal, and it does not mean she no longer needs you or is not attracted to you.

DID YOU KNOW?

If you haven't already, you will probably be given the option to see a genetic counselor at or around the time of the first prenatal appointment. Genetic counselors ask you many questions about your family's medical history and may also take blood and tissue samples from both you and your partner to find out if either of you has specific genes that carry diseases such as cystic fibrosis, sickle cell anemia, and Tay-Sachs—all three of which both parents must carry in order for it to be passed on to your baby.

One way to increase the physical closeness between you and your partner is to give her massages a few times a week. This is an excellent way to pamper her and get some skin-on-skin time. Consider surprising her with fresh sheets, massage oil, and soft music. Treat her as though she is special and to be adored—from head to toe. Start by rubbing her shoulders and work your way down her body to her back, legs, and feet. Spending just 20 or 30 minutes touching your partner's body increases her blood flow and dramatically reduces stress and muscle tension. As a result, she will be more open to sexual intimacy and general physical closeness.

Of course, not everyone has the time or energy to give a full body massage several times a week, so you'll have to find other ways to create intimacy through physical contact. A more subtle way of dealing with mom's distance is to use the "hands on" approach. Whenever you are in the same room, let your hand rest lightly on some part of her body. For example, if she is doing dishes, place your hand on the small of her back as you talk. When walking, clasp her hand for a few minutes. Let your arm wrap around her shoulder in the movie theater, and place your hand on her knee during dinner.

Above all, always remember to hold her when you kiss her "hello" and "goodbye." And give her more than a peck on the cheek! Studies show deep kissing releases the stress-relieving hormone oxytocin, and that men who kiss their partners every day live an average of 5 years longer than those who don't. Besides, kissing often leads to other methods of physical closeness that can reel your partner in and make you feel like a couple again.

HOW DAD CAN HELP

During the second month, your partner will start to experience a few to all of the pregnancy symptoms. As a result she will feel sick, tired, and cranky most of the time. You will probably get pretty tired of having to be in "sympathy" mode all the time. When you feel like you just can't sympathize any more, try to imagine what it's like to be in her body. Realizing how genuinely uncomfortable pregnancy is can help mitigate the frustration you feel.

Ways to help her out include:

Take on chores that exacerbate mom's back pain: With all of the movement going on in mom's pelvic area, she is likely to have moderate to severe back pain. By doing the vacuuming, changing the sheets, and carrying laundry and groceries, you can help to minimize her misery.

Make a family dental appointment: Dental care during pregnancy is important to preventing gum disease and tooth decay. During pregnancy, excess blood circulation causes mom's gums to swell and bleed. This makes her susceptible to bacteria that

Mom can become prone to hemorrhoids while she is pregnant. One reason is that high levels of progesterone cause the outer part of the veins to relax, which allows them to swell. If your partners is troubled by hemorrhoids, try adding more fiber to her diet to make bowel movements easier, since straining can result in hemorrhoids. She should also get plenty of exercise, as the increased blood circulation can prevent blood from pooling in the lower half of the body—another reason why veins tend to swell.

can cause infection. Head off trouble by offering to make dentist appointments for the both of you.

Be wary of touching her breasts: Your partner's breasts have probably never looked so good to you. Rounder, fuller breasts are one of the better physical signs of pregnancy. But the owner of those breasts is feeling a lot of pain and soreness in that area. Therefore, be careful of accidentally brushing mom's breasts while in bed or around the house. Also, let her know that "you heard" wearing a soft-cup sports bra to bed minimizes pain during sleep.

If she's hot, you're hot: Mom's body is heating up as hormones, blood production, and her metabolism increase. So, even though you may be freezing, let her run the air conditioning in winter if she needs to. Just throw on a sweatshirt and smile.

Let her sleep in: Mom's body is undergoing a complete overhaul, which is an exhausting process. Let her sleep in, take naps, and go to bed early without hassle. To make getting her required rest easier, record shows that run late, make plans for late afternoon

ⓘ PREGNANCY FACT

Braxton-Hicks are uterine contractions that can start as early as 6 weeks into pregnancy. Mom won't be able to feel them yet, but down the road, she may start to notice a slight sensation of tightening and releasing in her lower abdomen. Some women feel them as early as the second trimester, though they are more common during the third. If your partner experiences Braxton-Hicks contractions with any intensity before 37 weeks, however, you should immediately let your doctor know.

or early evening, and be willing to take the couch if your snoring wakes her during the night.

Use aromatherapy to help quell nausea: Anyone who has ever had the stomach flu knows how unbearable just one hour of nausea and vomiting can be. Now imagine feeling that way for 3 months or more! Pregnancy sickness will wear your partner down and cause her a great deal of misery. You can help by learning how to use scents that trick the brain away from feeling nauseous. Examples include lemon, peppermint, lavender, ginger, and grapefruit. These are effective when used fresh, in candles, teas, or essential oils. In oil form they can be burned in a diffuser or used in the bath and during massage—but oils should never be ingested by your partner as they can be harmful to baby's development.

HOW DAD CAN BE INVOLVED

One way for dad to be involved at this stage of pregnancy is to know when symptoms exceed what is normal. This can present a particular challenge to first-time parents who tend to panic over every little symptom. If ever in doubt, always err on the side of caution and call your healthcare provider. But learning to distinguish what symptoms are normal and which indicate a problem can help you be the voice of reason during a very unreasonable time.

Call the doctor if your partner experiences:

- Vaginal bleeding—more than spotting
- Chunks of tissue in toilet or underwear
- Abdominal pain
- Fever of 102 degrees or higher
- Sudden and excessive swelling of her hands, feet, or face
- Severe headache
- Involuntary shaking
- Gushing fluid from her vagina
- Change in vision
- Unable to keep food or liquid down for more than 24 hours
- Severe and frequent vomiting—more than 3 times a day
- Pain during urination
- Inability to urinate
- Constipation lasting more than 3 days
- Chest pain
- A fall or car accident
- Fainting or severe dizziness

DAD'S RESPONSIBILITIES

Now is a good time to take a hard look at your finances and come up with a budget for after your baby is born. Having a baby can be financially stressful if you are not prepared for the associated costs. According to BabyCenter LLC, the first year of life costs parents $7,542 in gear, diapers, clothes, and other essentials. You can plan to spend another $125,000 to $250,000 until your child turns 18—and more if you plan to help with college tuition. Taking

✖ FOOD FOR THOUGHT

Consider steaming, blending, and then freezing a large batch of broccoli puree to add nutrition to sauces, baked goods, and salads. There may come a point when mom's nausea prevents her from eating this powerhouse vegetable, and so disguising it in other foods is a great way to reap the nutritional benefits. Broccoli contains vitamins C, K, A, E, B1, B3, B5, as well as folate, fiber, protein, iron, calcium, and omega 3s. You can be helpful by serving mom foods with broccoli puree mixed in.

on the responsibility of figuring out where this money will come from allows mom to spend this time focusing on her health. Also, focusing on finances allows you to sink your teeth into something that requires attention, thought, detail, and planning. In other words, it will keep you busy when you have no idea what to do with yourself!

First, think about your current spending habits. Keep receipts for everything you and your partner purchase—from candy bars to big ticket items—and add the total up at the end of the month. Pay attention to whether you use cash or credit and if your spending frequently exceeds your income. If so, you have some serious work to do. Once you evaluate your spending habits, establish a monthly budget and stick to it. Continue to collect receipts for accuracy and keep tabs on spontaneous purchases. These impulse buys add up and can devastate your "baby budget."

For men who are already fiscally conservative, this may not be a big life change. For those who are used to at-will spending, establishing a baby budget can feel stifling and frustrating. It is also the first sign that Life is Really About to Change. It is normal to feel resistant to these changes. But after awhile, you will get used to the idea—and even be proud of—the job of financially providing for your family.

"A baby is God's opinion that life should go on."
~ Carl Sandburg

Notes . . . .

Lunar Month

Three

First Trimester

Lunar Month three · · · · · · · · ·

MONTHLY TO-DO LISTS

- ❑ Help mom manage morning sickness using aromatherapy
- ❑ Be your partner's sounding board for fears, excitement, concerns, etc.
- ❑ Take on additional chores
- ❑ Encourage non-pregnancy interests and hobbies for you and your partner
- ❑ Discuss with your partner when to share the big news, and with whom
- ❑ Research the ins and outs of your insurance plan
- ❑ Help your partner get enough iodine to support your baby's developing thyroid gland. Iodine is found in sea vegetables (like kelp), yogurt, milk, eggs, mozzerella cheese, and strawberries.
- ❑ Expand your pregnancy vocabulary

MY PERSONAL CHECKLIST:

- ❑ ....
- ❑ ....
- ❑ ....

MY HOPES FOR THIS MONTH:

....
....
....
....
....
....
....
....
....

What's Happening: Mom & Baby

First Trimester

WHAT'S HAPPENING TO MOM

Mom's anatomy continues to change as her body is transformed into a life support system for two. While "under construction," she may experience an increase in certain symptoms—such as shortness of breath—or be lucky enough to see some side effects—like the need to pee every 30 minutes—subside. Whatever her pregnancy experience so far, it is likely that she will suffer from at least a few symptoms before month's end.

One such symptom is increased fatigue and possibly anemia. As her circulatory system undergoes significant expansion, her heart beats faster per minute and must increase its blood production. This may cause the early development of varicose veins to bulge in her legs, vagina, or breasts. Though she may find them unsightly, they are harmless and a sign that her veins are making room for the extra blood. Also, your partner may develop anemia if she does not get enough iron in her diet. Therefore, she should drink plenty of water and eat iron-rich foods, such as liver, beans, sardines, pumpkin seeds, and leafy greens. Pay close attention to her level of fatigue, as it may be a side effect of anemia.

- Intense nausea
- Fatigue
- Frequent urination or slight relief from pressure on the bladder
- Constipation
- Heartburn
- Headaches
- Dizziness
- Increased appetite
- Aversions to foods and/or certain smells
- Bulging veins
- Anxious to make it to the second trimester
- Shortness of breath
- Anemia

The additional stress put on her circulatory system may cause mom to feel out of breath. To support placental and fetal growth and move enough oxygen to mom's organs, her lungs must increase their capacity to take in 30 to 40 percent more air with each breath. Even so, pressure from other organs and a faster heartbeat may cause her to feel as though she cannot get good, deep breaths. This can lead to anxiety. Help your partner relax, breathe, and know that this is a normal side effect that will subside in the third trimester.

This month, mom should be eating an additional 300 calories a day to provide energy and essential nutrients to both her and baby. The majority of these calories should be from healthy, fresh foods. Eating well will decrease the severity of symptoms such as indigestion and sugar-rushes that can exacerbate feeling out of breath and tired. Moreover, a bland diet free of fatty, greasy, or spicy foods will decrease nausea and heartburn.

Something else to consider is that increases of the pregnancy hormone progesterone cause the smooth muscles of your partner's digestive tract to relax. Thus, food takes much longer to break down, and moves through the digestive process more slowly. While this gives baby more time to absorb the nutrients in mom's blood, it also makes mom more prone to heartburn. In addition, high levels of progesterone can cause mom to feel dizzy—the hormone allows blood to reach the fetus, but slows the return of blood back up to mom's brain. First thing in the morning is a common time for pregnant women to feel dizzy. If she ever faints, call the doctor to check in. Fainting can be normal or a sign that something is wrong. Assuming everything is fine, managing light-headedness can be as simple as mom stabilizing her blood sugar, getting enough rest, and staying well-hydrated.

Some time this month your partner may also experience increased pain in her pelvic region. This is caused by the stretching of the ligaments that are attached to her uterus. Getting up too fast after sitting or lying down can send mom back into her chair, doubled over in pain. It can be scary to witness, but it is normal. She just needs to take her time when moving in ways that tug on these ligaments. She may also feel a stabbing pain when coughing or sneezing. She can help stabilize her muscles by pressing her lower back into a wall when she feels a cough or a sneeze coming on. These pains will likely increase as her uterus continues to grow up and out of the pelvic area. If lower abdominal pain is ever accompanied by fever, chills, or bleeding, call the doctor right away. Otherwise, some lower abdominal discomfort is completely normal and to be expected throughout pregnancy.

As the first trimester draws to a close, it is common for women to get a break from the urgent need to pee. This happens as mom's uterus moves slightly higher in her pelvis, reducing pressure on the bladder. However, progesterone will relax the tubes that carry urine from the kidneys to the bladder, making mom feel like she is never quite empty. One way for her to deal with this is to lean forward

> ## ⓘ PREGNANCY FACT
>
> When it comes to food safety, it can literally be a matter of life and death for your baby. Thus, to avoid bacterium called listeria monocyotogenes, the FDA recommends that pregnant women avoid eating hot dogs, smoked or raw seafood, unpasteurized dairy products, and soft cheeses. It is also recommended that all perishable foods be stored at or below 40 degrees. If mom contracts the bacteria, it can lead to an infection called listeriosis, which can lead to miscarriage or still-birth.

while on the toilet to "squeeze" every drop of urine out. If you're not comfortable sharing this tip with her, you can mark this page and leave it in a conspicuous place (like the bathroom!) for her to find.

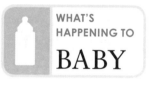

WHAT'S HAPPENING TO BABY

The third month of pregnancy is one of explosive development for baby. He will start to lengthen and put on weight, becoming close to 4 inches long. By the end of week 12, he is about the size of a nectarine.

This month, your baby's kidneys will start to produce urine. This sterile fluid becomes part of the amniotic fluid and causes its volume to increase. In addition to adding a protective cushion around the fetus, amniotic fluid is measured by your partner's doctor to judge whether baby's kidneys are functioning properly. Meanwhile, his intestines are slowly moving out of the umbilical cord and into his abdomen.

In another exciting development, your baby's external sex organs will form by the end of the month. Though it may not yet be visible on an ultrasound, your son's tiny penis will protrude from his pubic area as his prostate gland develops. If you are expecting a daughter, her vaginal folds are forming as her ovaries—which already contain approximately 2 million eggs—start to move down into her pelvis. Additionally, your baby's thyroid gland forms this month and begins producing hormones that will eventually regulate his or her metabolism.

**WHAT TO
EXPECT
DR.S VISITS**

Certain tests are performed at each checkup, with some new additions as the pregnancy progresses. With some exceptions, all tests are optional and your doctor should respect your decision to pass on tests you do not think are necessary. However, depending on your age and medical history, you should give serious consideration to each test that is offered before turning it down.

🔍 **DID YOU KNOW?**

The fundus is the opening at the top of the uterus that is opposite the cervix. When you visit your doctor each month for your prenatal checkup, he will press his hand gently into mom's lower abdomen to find the fundus, and measure from it to the top of the pubic bone. This measurement helps determine if your baby is on-target with his growth. Measurement of the fundus can help identify problems in the pregnancy if the growth is deemed too little or too much when compared with the gestational age of your baby.

+ HEALTH CONCERNS

If mom was treated for depression before she became pregnant, now is not the time to stop her treatment plan. It is true that if she is taking antidepressants for mild depression, your doctor may advise her to go off them while pregnant. However, women who suffer from major depression may be at higher risk for complications. The doctor may recommend that she continue taking antidepressants. Continue with therapy and be sure to keep your OB-GYN in the loop.

Physical exam and urine specimen: These reoccurring tests help keep tabs on mom and baby's overall health.

Doppler/heart monitor: At each appointment, you will have the opportunity to hear your baby's heartbeat amplified by a Doppler.

Chorionic villus sampling (CVS): Between the 8th and 11th week, your doctor will offer to perform CVS to determine whether your baby is at risk for certain developmental abnormalities, such as Down syndrome. The doctor inserts a thin tube through the cervix into the uterus. Fetal cells are removed and tested. If CVS reveals a predisposition toward birth defects, the doctor will recommend your partner have amniocentesis around week 16.

The First Trimester Screen: This combination blood test and ultrasound evaluates (but does not diagnose) the risk for developing chromosomal abnormalities. It is offered to moms between the 11th and 13th weeks of pregnancy. An abnormal test result means that further testing is necessary and does not necessarily indicate chromosomal defects.

What's Happening:
Dad

First Trimester

It is almost time to breathe a sigh of relief, dad, as your partner is nearly one-third of the way through her pregnancy. This is significant, because when the first trimester ends the odds of miscarriage drop to about 1 percent if the baby's heartbeat has been detected at the last prenatal appointment. Also, there is light at the end of the tunnel for mom—and thereby for dad—since this should be the last month during which nausea is a crushing symptom.

WHAT DAD IS THINKING AND FEELING

By now you might be thinking, "I had no idea pregnancy could be so emotionally draining—for me!" Indeed, it is possible that at this point in the pregnancy you are feeling a little resentful about your increasingly demanding role as your partner's support person, work horse, and occasional whipping boy. It is normal to have days when it feels downright impossible to navigate her irrational demands. Take a minute to acknowledge your frustration, know it is normal, and then remind yourself that you can take a break from this situation at any time—whereas your partner is trapped in her body with uncomfortable symptoms for the next several months. Looking at the situation in this way can help you to gain some perspective and keep your patience over the next 6 or 7 months.

Meanwhile, when you and your partner take a break from the frequent outbursts, arguments, and squabbles that often plague expecting couples, take the opportunity to tell your partner how proud you are of her. Let her know that you are amazed by her body's ability to support and house your baby—and that you see her as remarkable for being able to shoulder so many adverse symptoms at once. You may be surprised how far a little praise will go in diffusing a volatile situation. And if she ends up in tears, well, at least this time they are tears of joy and appreciation!

THINGS DAD SHOULD KNOW

Continue to learn and use the vocabulary of pregnancy. Doing so will help you stay informed and keep up with your partner and her doctor at prenatal visits.

This month, learn and understand the following important pregnancy-related concepts and terms:

Areola: The darker-colored ring that surrounds the nipple. As pregnancy progresses, this pigmentation will become darker.

Amniocentesis: Test performed where amniotic fluid is removed from the amniotic sac with a large needle. Fluid is then screened for genetic defects.

Cervix: The opening at the base of the uterus

Chloasma (or Melasma): Darkening of the pigmentation on the face caused by pregnancy hormones. Also known as the "mask of pregnancy," this phenomenon causes brown patches to appear on mom's face that will darken with sun exposure.

HEALTH CONCERNS

Some pregnant women find that drinking liquids makes them feel ill. If mom has trouble drinking, be sure she eats foods that contain water, like fruits and squash. It is also helpful to drink water, milk, or juice between meals instead of during. Fluids with food tend to increase nausea, bloating, and discomfort. Saving her daily servings of low-fat drinks and water for between meals will increase the likelihood of it staying down. Alert your doctor right away if she is consistently too nauseous to keep liquid down.

Fetus: An unborn baby from 10 weeks until birth

Fundus: The top of the uterus. Doctors measure the distance between the pelvis and the top of the fundus to help determine the due date.

Hemorrhoids: Swollen veins in and around the rectum caused by increased blood flow pumping through mom's body during pregnancy

Intrauterine growth restriction (IUGR): Stunted growth of the fetus during gestation

Linea nigra: A dark line that appears during pregnancy. It runs from mom's pubic area to her belly button.

Placenta Previa: When the placenta develops in such a way that it covers the opening of the cervix

Placental abruption: When the placenta is prematurely separated from the uterus

Umbilical cord: A thick, rope-like cord that connects baby to the placenta. The umbilical cord transfers waste products away from the baby and ushers in nutrients and oxygen.

Varicose veins: Swollen or dilated blood vessels

Vena cava: A major vein that sends deoxygenized blood into the right atrium of the heart. Women are encouraged to sleep on their left sides during pregnancy to avoid putting too much weight on this vein, which obstructs blood flow.

HELPFUL HINTS FOR DAD

As the first trimester comes to an end, it is time to become intimately familiar with your medical insurance plan. Do not let another day go by without knowing exactly what your medical insurance plan covers and how much money you are responsible for paying after the birth of your baby.

The following questions will help you determine whether your insurance coverage is adequate for this major life change:

What type of medical insurance plan do we have? HMOs are one kind of common plan. Short for healthcare maintenance organization, HMOs are prepaid health plans that usually focus on preemptive care that is limited to the HMO-specified network. Patients are required to select a primary care physician and pay a co-pay for doctor visits. Co-pays are also required upon admittance to the hospital during labor and delivery. HMOs can be

---

🔍 **DID YOU KNOW?**

Many pregnant women have vivid dreams when they are expecting—particularly during the first trimester. It is theorized that hormone surges are responsible for this sleep-cinema. In fact, many women report that they dreamed they were pregnant before they ever took a test, and even more pregnant women claim to have dreamed their baby's gender very early on. Urge your partner to write her dreams down. Keeping a pregnancy dream journal is cathartic and an incredible keepsake to pass down to your child.

---

cost-effective but frustrating as choice of doctors and hospitals are strictly limited by the approved network.

Another common plan is the POS. Short for point of service, POS plans are similar to HMOs, but coverage is extended to out-of-network services with a referral from your primary care physician. Patients may also self-refer, but this increases out-of-pocket cost, sometimes significantly.

Finally, there are PPOs. Short for preferred provider organizations, PPOs are similar to HMO and POS plans in that you must choose a primary care doctor. However, you may also see any doctor outside of the network and still receive some coverage. Patients are often required to meet a deductible before insurance picks up the tab, and thereafter patients may still be responsible for a co-pay or coinsurance percentage.

Reading can reduce stress and improve cognitive functioning. This can help you and your partner get a handle on her forgetfulness, better known as "pregnancy brain." Switch back and forth between reading silently and reading aloud so your baby can get used to hearing your voice. This is also a great way to bond with your partner— read a few pages of a book to her belly each night. Keep track of the books you read and why you chose them—it will be fun to revisit this in a few years.

How familiar are you with the following insurance terms?

Coinsurance: the amount of money you are responsible for paying after meeting your deductible. For example, after paying your $250 deductible for the first 2 prenatal visits, you may become responsible for 20 percent of the cost of subsequent visits while the insurance company picks up the other 80 percent.

Co-pay: the fee you pay each time you see your doctor or purchase a prescription. For example, your partner may have a $25 co-pay for each prenatal visit and a $250 co-pay for admittance to the hospital. This fee should cover all costs related to labor and delivery.

Covered expenses: the services and fees that insurance will cover. Do not assume that everything related to pregnancy is covered! For example, your insurance may cover certain types of medications that are used during labor and delivery but not others. Not knowing what expenses are covered can become a very expensive lesson in reading the fine print of your insurance policies.

Exclusions: services and fees the insurance company will not cover.

Maximum out-of-pocket expenses: This is a number chosen by the insurance company that promises your cost for a particular year will not exceed a certain amount. For example, your policy may state you will not be responsible for more than $1,500 for the year, including deductibles and co-insurance fees.

Pre-existing condition: a heath condition that existed or occurred prior to the start of coverage. Find out if any health problems your partner developed before coverage began are covered under your insurance plan.

Evaluate the strength of your insurance plan by asking some additional questions of your insurance provider and human resources representative, such as:

- What kind of coverage do I have?
- How comprehensive is my plan?
- What are the maternity benefits?
- What prenatal tests are covered?
- Does our plan offer maternity classes?
- How many prenatal visits are paid for by the insurance company?
- How do I file claims?
- What are the hospitalization benefits?
- Does our preferred healthcare provider accept our insurance?
- What coverage is offered for high-risk pregnancy?
- Is Cesarean delivery covered under the plan?
- What labor and delivery medications are covered?
- Is my partner's choice of anesthesia limited by our coverage?
- Does our insurance specify the length of hospital stay covered?
- How do I add our baby to the plan?

> ### ⓘ PREGNANCY FACT
>
> Approximately 3 percent of women are pregnant with twins each year—and the numbers are increasing as more moms are aided by fertility drugs. Twins are conceived in one of two ways: Fraternal twins develop when two separate eggs are fertilized by two separate sperm and implanted in the uterus, while identical twins form from the same divided egg. Fraternal twins are as genetically similar to each other as they are to any other siblings, while identical twins have identical genetic composition.

- Can we choose our pediatrician?
- How much time do we have after baby is born to add her to our policy?

Once you know the ins and outs of your insurance plan you can make informed decisions about choosing doctors, where to deliver, and whether to use certain medications based on what you can afford.

COMMON QUESTIONS THAT DADS HAVE

In addition to medical coverage, you may also have questions about other types of insurance. Keep in mind that there is no shortage of insurance plans out there and not all of them are necessary for parents-to-be. So though you may feel pressured by your insurance carrier to add them, do your homework before purchasing any additional policies.

Start by considering the most common questions dads have about additional insurance coverage:

Do I need life insurance for my child? The short answer is no. Life insurance is designed to replace some portion of lost income in the event an earner dies. Since your baby will be detracting from your income and not earning any, there is no reason to take out a life insurance plan for her.

Should I add accidental death insurance if I often travel for work? The answer depends on your own assessment of your risk that you will die in an accident. If you have a dangerous job, drive long distances, and fly enough to be concerned, it may be worth it. But since the chance of dying an accidental death is very slim, this insurance is not one that should be at the top of your list.

Can my partner use disability insurance? This question can only be answered by your partner's employer. In many cases, benefits may kick in if mom becomes seriously ill during pregnancy

+ HEALTH CONCERNS

Mom's feet and ankles may swell this trimester, especially when she sits for long stretches. This condition is called edema and is due to poor circulation and fluid that pools in the bottom of the legs and ankles. A great solution is for her to invest in a good pair of compression hose. Compression hose work by putting a gradual amount of pressure from the ankles (most pressure) up the leg (least pressure), increasing the flow of blood back up to the upper half of her body, thus relieving leg cramps and swelling.

DID YOU KNOW?

Traveling while your partner is pregnant is fine as long as you have the OK from your doctor. Most women feel better in their second trimester, so it might behoove you to wait until she is 15 or 16 weeks along before you take a trip. Keep in mind that no matter how you get where you are going—by car or plane—mom should move her body as often as she can, even if she just makes circles with her feet or walks up and down the airplane aisle. This will help prevent fluid accumulation in her ankles and feet.

and has to stop working. Other companies do not allow coverage until after baby is born. Encourage your partner to find out how her employer manages disability insurance for pregnancy.

When should I add my child as a beneficiary to my life insurance policy? You should be able to add your child as a beneficiary at any time. However, if you want to up your coverage you may be subjected to a health evaluation that increases your premium.

Is renter's insurance worth the cost? Considering that the average cost of renter's insurance in America is $12 per month or $240 a year, yes. This cost covers up to $30,000 worth of damage. However, read the fine print regarding "Acts of God," such as flooding, storm damage, tornadoes, earthquakes, and fires, because these are often excluded in high-risk areas.

HOW DAD CAN DEAL

At some point during the pregnancy it is common for men to develop symptoms similar to those experienced by mom. In fact up to 90 percent of men experience sympathetic pregnancy symptoms, called couvade, at some point during the third month. Symptoms of couvade are nearly identical to those of your partner: nausea, headaches, cravings, aversions, weight gain or loss, mood swings, and even nosebleeds. In addition, men who live with their pregnant partners can experience shifts in hormone levels, just like mom. Researchers who study this phenomenon note that symptoms tend to completely disappear shortly after baby is born and mom feels better.

Even if you do not experience this extreme version of sympathetic pregnancy, odds are you are having a physical reaction to the pregnancy at least some of the time. Living with a woman whose body is being transformed by pregnancy is powerful and, to some degree, contagious. Thus, it is normal to feel nauseous while in her presence or to get headaches. These symptoms can also be attributed to the stress of trying to organize your life to receive a new family member.

Learning to control your stress level is just as important to your health as it is to mom's. Just as her pregnancy symptoms are contagious, so too, is your stress. If you come home from work hollering about how there is no way to afford the baby, her symptoms are likely to worsen, over time even threatening her and the baby's health. So it's important to sort out what exactly is making you stressed. Start by making a list of fears and concerns about having a baby. Take your list to a trusted friend or relative—preferably someone who is also a father—and sit back as he explains how he felt exactly the same as you do now. Discuss solutions, or just talk and listen. Merely sharing the experience is often enough to release the stress that has built up so far. Also, get lots of exercise. Try running, swimming, walking, or biking, or join a team sport, such as basketball or soccer. As long as it doesn't meet so often that it takes you excessively away from your partner, the physical expression of energy, combined with camaraderie and team focus, can greatly reduce many manly symptoms related to your partner's pregnancy.

HOW DAD CAN HELP

Your partner may be going through a major "I hate the way I look" phase. This can be attributed to a pale, broken-out complexion and a slight weight gain. Since she probably does not yet look pregnant, she may worry others think she is just getting fat, especially if no one else knows she is pregnant. In addition, she is feeling quite bloated these days thanks to water retention and constipation. She may even have dark circles under her eyes due to lack of sleep, which will make her feel like no amount of makeup will improve them. Tell her that you love and cherish her appearance, no matter what changes she is going through, and remind her that many of her worst symptoms are temporary.

Perhaps the greatest help you can be to your partner this month is to boost her self-esteem as it gets flushed down the toilet with her breakfast every morning. Help her gain perspective on her appearance. Remember that no matter how good or bad she actually looks, her mind's eye is a devastating critic. Start each day by giving her compliments that are true. Examples include telling her she is brave, courageous, beautiful, and strong. The flow of these words together creates a picture she cannot refute. And by mixing physical compliments with ones about her personality and character, you downplay the importance of superficial prettiness and emphasize her beauty as a whole person.

If mom is suffering from pregnancy-related symptoms, try acupuncture. Studies show that acupuncture can offer relief from many of the side effects and symptoms of pregnancy. One study showed that acupuncture during the first trimester significantly reduced morning sickness and severe vomiting when participants received regular treatments. In the second trimester, women saw relief from hemorrhoids, heartburn, and headaches. In the third trimester, women experienced a decrease in aches and pains.

In addition, encourage her to buy clothes that fit. Tell her there is no shame in gaining weight while pregnant and that going up a size is a good sign. Let her know that you find her curves and increasing bust size sexy, and prove it by touching her often. Then let her go shopping and to a day spa to pamper herself. Hopefully, she will return feeling refreshed and pretty. If all of your efforts fail, consider mentioning your partner's sinking mood to her doctor. It is possible that she is depressed and may benefit from therapy—especially if she was diagnosed with the condition prior to getting pregnant.

Experiencing some degree of feeling down when pregnant is very common. Surging hormones, persistent negative symptoms, and lack of sleep can devastate the most even-tempered personalities. If this is the case, and your partner is not suffering from a more serious case of depression, just let her be. Allow her to experience her feelings without trying to talk her out of them. If crying actually helps her feel better, let her cry. As psychiatrist Francis J. Braceland once said, "The sorrow which has no vent in tears may make other organs weep."

> ### ⓘ PREGNANCY FACT
>
> Make mom an appointment for an evaluation with her dentist at least once while she is expecting. During pregnancy, hormones cause her gums to swell, and they may even split and bleed during a meal or when she brushes her teeth. Gums also become more vulnerable to bacteria and plaque, gingivitis, and even periodontitis, which can lead to low birth weight or premature delivery. As with everything, prevention is the best defense, so have her limit sweets, brush and floss after meals, and get plenty of calcium and vitamin C.

HOW DAD CAN BE INVOLVED

One way to get involved in the pregnancy this month is to discuss with your partner when to share the news with everyone else. Consider if there is a pecking order within your circles of family and friends. Who absolutely needs to know? Who might you not want to tell yet? People who are close to you and your partner should hear the news either in person or on the telephone. For those outside of your close-knit circle, it is fine to send emails or mass announcements.

Your pecking order might look something like this:
Parents: You and your partner's parents should definitely be told first. Preferably, at the same time. So, invite all of the parents over for dinner (or call them on conference call) to share the great news. The grandparents-to-be will appreciate being told in person and before the general public.

Siblings: If you or your partner has sisters, tell them next. Sisters usually cannot wait to hear this news! Immediately after calling sisters, share the news with any brothers in the family. Above all, avoid letting any siblings hear the news from your parents.

Friends: It is not required that you tell everyone in the phone book you are pregnant, but your intimate circle of friends should be high on your list. If there is a friend in your group who cannot keep a secret, tell her last so she doesn't beat you to the punch of sharing your exciting news with others.

Work: Sharing the news at work is definitely the trickiest community to deal with. You may wonder who is genuinely happy for you and who smiles as they plot taking over your projects and clients. If you tell anyone at work this month, tell your boss. He or she will need to know so you can come up for a game plan to manage your duties while you are on leave. Wait as long as possible to let other coworkers in on the secret to avoid scheming and behind-the-back talk.

Everyone else: Acquaintances, old friends, long-lost relatives, and your dog's veterinarian are low on the information totem pole. If the news spills out, fine, but do not feel pressured to tell everyone you've ever come in contact with that you are going to be a dad.

Once you've made a list of priority people, sit down with your partner and discuss your information dissemination plan. Make it fun by drawing graphs, pie charts, and family trees. Joke about how you think people might react and bring serious consideration to the table when it comes to telling employers.

✖ FOOD FOR THOUGHT

Consider adding sweet potatoes to your partner's pregnancy diet. Not only are they versatile and delicious, but they are full of important nutrients. Sweet potatoes contain proteins with antioxidant properties and are classified as an "antidiabetic" food. This means sweet potatoes have been shown to stabilize blood-sugar levels and decrease insulin resistance. Sweet potatoes are also a powerhouse for nutrients. Just one serving is packed with vitamin A, C, B6, as well as copper, dietary fiber, potassium, and iron.

DAD'S RESPONSIBILITIES

Your responsibility this month is to take stock of the changes your relationship has already undergone and prepare for more as baby's due date gets closer. Some of the changes you may have already noticed might seem more like losses: shorter periods of free time you both have, fewer sexual encounters, and less money to devote to hobbies are three of the ways in which your relationship may have changed.

But just because things are changing does not mean they are becoming worse. Having a baby deepens the connection you have with your partner, turning you into teammates in a way you probably never dreamed was possible. Your discussions may have changed from debating politics to debating baby names, but these conversations are intimate and personal in a way that many people never get to experience.

Whether the majority of changes up to this point have been positive, negative, or neutral, it is important to be aware of them as they are happening so you do not wake up one day after the baby is born and wonder, "How did we get here?" Indeed, many couples amble through pregnancy and the early months of baby's life without noticing that not only is their relationship very different but that many of these changes are permanent. Avoid continental drift in your relationship by committing to stay on the same page with your partner, no matter what. Your commitment to each other will stay constant as life's other variables change.

"Babies are such a nice way to start people."
~ Don Herold

Notes . . . .

Lunar Month

Four

Second Trimester

Lunar Month four · · · · · · · · ·

MONTHLY TO-DO LISTS

- ❑ Expect your partner to gain about a pound a week
- ❑ Don't make fun of your partner's weight gain—attempts to lose weight can be dangerous for the baby
- ❑ Do the laundry
- ❑ Attend this month's prenatal appointment
- ❑ Ask your partner out on a date
- ❑ Avoid becoming the food police
- ❑ Check in with mom during the day to see how she is feeling
- ❑ Keep a pregnancy journal to share with your child
- ❑ Make a list of home-improvement projects to be completed before baby comes home
- ❑ Replace batteries in smoke detectors throughout your house
- ❑ Make sure your partner goes to the dentist
- ❑ Learn the basics of investing

MY PERSONAL CHECKLIST:

- ❑ ....
- ❑ ....
- ❑ ....

MY HOPES FOR THIS MONTH:

....
....
....
....
....
....
....
....
....

What's Happening: Mom & Baby

Lunar Month 4

Second Trimester

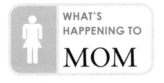

WHAT'S HAPPENING TO MOM

The second trimester is often considered the "honeymoon period" of pregnancy. It is so-called because for most women, the difficult symptoms—nausea and vomiting—start to wane. As a result, mom's appetite and energy levels increase, making her feel much better than she did just a week or two ago. However, a few new symptoms debut this month, such as congestion, nosebleeds, and forgetfulness. Though these symptoms are annoying, most moms prefer them to puking. By month's end, the pregnancy will become externally visible as mom develops a "baby bump" and sees a jump in her weight gain.

By the end of the fourth month, mom will have gained between 4 and 6 pounds, her cantaloupe-sized uterus will push up-and-out, and she will start to look pregnant. However, as this process unfolds, she may feel frustrated and sad that her clothes no longer fit. She might get emotional about her changing appearance, so it is important to reassure her that she is beautiful—and encourage her to buy clothes that fit.

Since nausea is on the decline, now is the time to get mom to fill up on all of the healthy foods she could not stomach during the

MOM'S Symptoms

- Constipation
- Decrease in nausea and vomiting
- Heartburn and gas
- Gingivitis and nosebleeds
- Vaginal discharge
- Yeast infections
- Hemorrhoids
- Varicose veins
- Darkening skin pigment
- Swelling of ankles
- Breast enlargement
- Forgetfulness
- Low self-esteem
- Increased energy level
- Pound-a-week weight gain
- "Baby bump" appears
- Congestion
- Cramp after orgasm

first trimester. The famous pregnancy appetite makes its debut this month. Though mom does not literally have to eat for 2, she may be hungry enough to try. It is especially important for her to make calories count, as she really only needs 300 extra per day. Having pre-portioned, healthy snacks at her fingertips, such as carrot and celery sticks, almonds, fruit, and yogurt, may help reduce her urge to binge on Doritos and banana splits.

Controlling those urges is important not only for mom's weight gain but also to maintaining her healthy gums and teeth. Indeed, due to increased blood volume, your partner's gums will swell and bleed this month. This leaves her vulnerable to gingivitis and bacterial infections. She'll want to limit sweets and brush often with a soft-bristled toothbrush. She may also notice an increase in other dental problems, such as the development of cavities. As baby grows and his bones harden, he will pull calcium from wherever he can get it—including from your partner's bones and teeth. Therefore, it is crucial that she consumes the recommended daily allowance of calcium (1,000 milligrams), which can reduce pregnancy-associated dental damage.

Increasing calcium intake often involves consuming more dairy products, which can exacerbate another symptom that develops around this time—congestion. Unfortunately, thanks to hormones, congestion and phlegm become a persistent issue this month. These are likely to last throughout the rest of the pregnancy. Your partner is likely to have a constant runny nose, along with post-nasal drip. These may drive her crazy and actually cause her nausea to flare up. Sudden congestion may also transform your partner into a roaring snorer. Running a cool-mist humidifier at night can help ease her breathing and help you both to get much-needed sleep. A humidifier can also help relieve the nosebleeds your partner may experience this month. These are a common side effect of increased estrogen production.

Pregnancy hormones might also cause your partner to develop yeast infections because they alter her delicate pH balance. Yeast infections are basically harmless but must be treated. Her doctor will likely recommend an over-the-counter treatment that will knock out the infection in 3 to 7 days. Avoid sex during this time. Yeast infections, in addition to being pretty gross, are contagious and can be passed back and forth.

If you could peer into your partner's uterus you would be amazed at what your baby is up to. Over the next several weeks, she will grow an additional 2 inches and react to outside stimuli. She'll develop the ability to swallow and constantly move her arms and legs.

One of the most important developments she makes this month is the accumulation of fat. This is important, because she'll need enough fat stored up when she is born to regulate her body

> Mom is trying to adjust to her new physique this trimester, and it may be hard for her (and maybe even you) to deal with. However, the fact is, gaining weight is a necessary part of pregnancy, and if she is gaining steadily, eating well, and exercising, then she should have little trouble getting back down to her pre-pregnancy weight and figure. Above all, pregnant women should never try to diet or lose weight. You can help by assuring mom that she is beautiful and sexy in her new body.

temperature and sustain her until mom's milk comes in. Fat will start to accumulate under her skin, which, at this point, is as thin and transparent as tracing paper.

Since her skin is still so thin, this month your baby starts to develop lanugo, a thin layer of fine hair that protects her outer layer. It keeps her warm in the womb and shields her from the perils of constant water-to-skin contact. Lanugo is not necessary after birth, so as she gets closer to her birthday the downy hair is shed into the amniotic fluid, digested, and turned into fat and meconium, which is your baby's first stool.

In addition to particles digested from the amniotic fluid, the calcium baby pulls from your partner's diet also contributes to her significant growth this month. As she absorbs calcium, your baby's bones gradually harden—or ossify—and her bone marrow matures. This, plus muscle development, gives your baby the uncontrollable urge to move. She'll be practicing a lot of new tricks, as she can now open and close her mouth to swallow and yawn and move her head side to side and up and down. She may even be able to do somersaults!

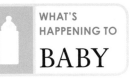

WHAT'S HAPPENING TO

BABY

If this is not your partner's first pregnancy, she may feel these first movements, called quickening. They'll feel similar to "butterflies" in the stomach. She may also notice that these flutters increase with outside stimuli, such as music, voices, or after eating spicy foods. This is because baby's nervous system is starting to specialize its duties—especially those of the five senses. Hearing is one of the first senses to become "tuned in" to the outside world. Therefore, this month is an excellent time to start reading, singing, and talking to her.

Finally, by the end of this month, her circulatory system is able to pump an impressive 25 to 30 quarts of blood through her tiny 6-inch, 7-ounce body. This is an important development with reassuring results: As your baby's heart gets stronger and more capable of

DID YOU KNOW?

Headaches are common during pregnancy for many reasons—hormones, caffeine withdrawal, congestion, and stress can all cause mild to severe headaches. As soon as your partner feels a headache coming on, take her to a dark room and put a soft ice pack on her head. Keep her well-hydrated, or have her sit in the bathroom while you run a hot shower. The steam will help break up the congestion and relieve pressure that causes headaches. Finally, Tylenol is approved to treat headaches for most pregnancies.

✚ HEALTH CONCERS

Exercising can sometimes cause slight uterine contractions. Though this can be scary, it is usually not cause for alarm. Many women fear they are in premature labor when they feel a tightening sensation in their lower abdomen, so it helps to know what premature labor actually is. It is signified by painful uterine contractions that don't stop after you've ceased exercising, or contractions accompanied by vaginal bleeding and/or a rush of discharge, cramping, backaches, and pelvic pressure.

handling increased blood volume, the risk for miscarriage and other problems are greatly reduced.

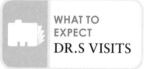 **WHAT TO EXPECT DR.S VISITS** Your partner will see her doctor for a routine checkup this month. The urine sample, physical, and Doppler monitor will feel routine to you now since this is most likely your third prenatal appointment. There is one new test this month that is optional, however—the triple and quadruple screening.

This one-time blood test allows your doctor to analyze AFP protein produced by your baby's liver. It also measures the hormones hCG and estriol (estrogen that is produced by the placenta instead of by the ovaries). The information gathered from this test can help your doctor detect neural tube and chromosomal disorders. Like all pregnancy diagnostics, results most often indicate that further testing is required rather than diagnose a specific problem. Curious results from this screening often cause doctors to suggest an amniocentesis for more information and clarification.

What's Happening: Dad

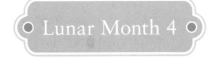

Lunar Month 4

Second Trimester

The fourth month is when dad gets to heave a great sigh of relief. For most moms, the second trimester is the "honeymoon period" which is marked by a significant decrease in the risk of miscarriage, the abatement of many symptoms, and an increase in energy level. Enjoy this window of relief and encourage your partner to indulge with you in spontaneity, fun, and travel during this special time.

WHAT DAD IS THINKING AND FEELING

At the beginning of this month you should be feeling relieved; by this point, your baby's statistical chance for survival has increased exponentially. Fathers-to-be are often overcome with relief upon learning that 80 percent of miscarriages occur by the 12th week of pregnancy, and that the chances of spontaneous abortion decreases with each passing week. This knowledge helps you relax a bit and offers you a chance to settle in to the reality of becoming a father. Believing that a baby is actually going to be living with you soon may inspire you to start preparations for his arrival.

You may also be feeling impressed with your partner, who is coming out of her first trimester fog. Feel free to tell her, "I don't know how you dealt with feeling sick for 10 weeks! You're amazing!" As the symptoms that clouded her mood and disposition these last few months slip away, you'll notice a happier, less fatigued, and more fun partner. Her increased energy also makes it a great time to take on baby-prep projects or indulge in occasional weekend getaways.

Because you are antsy for fun, you might find yourself becoming impatient with your partner's symptoms should they resurface. You may even doubt their intensity and think she is exaggerating to get attention or extra help with chores, or even that she is imagining it. Try and give her the benefit of the doubt—pregnancy is tough on her body in a way you will never truly know. Expand your empathy threshold by a couple of weeks and wait it out. If your partner truly does not feel any better by the middle of this month, talk to the doctor about potential causes and treatments. But if she is like most women, she will be ready to get back out into the world by the 14th week—and take you with her. Indeed, the onset of the second trimester is often when both mom and dad start to feel like a family instead of a couple.

THINGS DAD SHOULD KNOW

The following list of terms will be helpful to know at the start of the second trimester:

Alphafetoprotein (AFP): Protein produced and secreted by the fetal liver into mom's bloodstream. Abnormally high levels of AFP may indicate developmental problems, such as neural-tube defects, whereas low AFP may point to Down's syndrome.

Biophysical profile: Evaluates baby's health before birth

Braxton-Hicks contractions: The tightening and releasing of the uterus during pregnancy

Chadwick's sign: Purplish-blue coloring of the mucous

➕ HEALTH CONCERNS

Many moms-to-be turn to artificial sweeteners to cut down on sugar intake. However, there is not enough research available to know what effects they have on babies in utero. Scientists advise pregnant women against ingesting saccharin, as there is evidence it can potentially increase baby's risk for bladder cancer. Aspartame, a more common sweetener, is considered safe in small amounts, but it is advisable to limit mom's intake of the sugar substitute as there are conflicting reports about its safety when used regularly.

membranes of the cervix and vagina during pregnancy

Colostrum: Yellow-colored fluid that leaks from the breast before mom's milk comes in. May be present as early as the second trimester, but is most often seen at the end of the third.

Diastasis recti: Painful condition when mom's abdominal muscles become separated as the pregnancy progresses and pushes her belly out

Fetal goiter: The development of an oversized thyroid in a fetus

Gestational diabetes: Pregnancy-induced metabolic condition that results in diabetes. This condition is cured once baby and placenta are delivered.

Group-B streptococcal infection (GBS): Bacterial infection that can be found in a pregnant woman's vagina or rectum that can be harmful to baby during a vaginal delivery

Incompetent cervix: A cervix that dilates, or opens, without contractions too early in pregnancy

Preeclampsia: Condition that includes high blood pressure and severe edema. May precede eclampsia, a dangerous, potentially life-threatening condition marked by seizures and possible coma.

Pruritis gravidarum: A condition signified by constant itching that develops during pregnancy

Quickening: Feeling baby move for the first time

Restless leg syndrome (RLS): Condition in which women experience a tingling, creepy-crawling, or cramping sensation of the legs, particularly when trying to rest or sleep. Up to 20 percent of pregnant women develop RLS.

HELPFUL HINTS FOR DAD

At this point, many dads-to-be find themselves obsessing over a particular question: How am I going to support a family? Even with mom employed, this question sits heavily on the minds of dads everywhere. Though more women are going back to work sooner after having a baby, men are still viewed as the breadwinners. Another reason is that for the average American, two incomes simply are not enough to support one or more children until their 18th birthday without going into at least some debt. Indeed, according to the U.S. Census Bureau, the median household income is $49,800. After paying for housing, taxes, food, transportation, and other expenses, there is little left over to save for retirement or college funds. Since it is unlikely that you or your partner will be able to earn significantly more money or take on another job with a new baby on the way, you

DID YOU KNOW?

Some parents can't wait to find out their baby's sex so they can begin choosing names and designing the nursery. Others prefer to wait until the birth to learn the sex. If you're dying to find out your baby's sex, it is possible around this time to tell by ultrasound. However, it is still early in the pregnancy, thus there is a certain amount of error possible when deciphering the baby's sex in this way. If you are scheduled for an amniocentesis, though, this test will be able to tell with accuracy whether you are carrying a boy or a girl.

have to get creative with your budget and learn to invest.

Investing can be scary for those who are new to it. In fact, many people view investing the way they do gambling: an unnecessary risk. Though there is some risk involved with investing, it is not like going to a casino and betting on a game of Blackjack. Rather, investing is a way to put your money to work for you. This does not guarantee you will become wealthy, but is a useful, even necessary tool to add to your existing finances and increase your financial security over time.

The fourth month is the perfect time to learn about the different kinds of investments you can make. Below you will find basic information about the most popular types. Once your learn the basics, continue the investing process with your employer, a financial advisor, or brokerage firm. These are professionals who will encourage you to have a well-rounded portfolio and advise you based on your particular financial situation.

Sodium is a necessary mineral for pregnant women to help regulate their body fluids. Thus, mom should not go on a low-sodium diet. However, there is a difference between sodium and salt. Table salt is only 40 percent sodium, and should be limited. Sodium found naturally in foods is an important component of the pregnancy diet. Be sure to read food labels and keep in mind that your partner should consume around 2,400 milligrams of sodium each day while pregnant and nursing.

Bonds: When you purchase a bond, you are buying part of a government or corporation's debt. Bonds are low-risk, low-reward investments, but you are virtually guaranteed to get your money back, plus interest. Interest payments are fixed and issued once or twice a year. The full loan is repaid when it reaches maturity— such as in 1, 5, 10, or 30 years.

Stocks: Purchasing stock in a company makes you a shareholder, or part owner. This entitles you to a percentage of the company's earnings, called dividends. However, the stock market fluctuates, and it is very possible you will never see dividends for a particular stock. The risk can be high—if a company loses value or goes under, your stock will plummet, and you will lose your money. But if the value of the stock rises, you can potentially earn a lot. Knowing which company to invest in and when to sell is difficult, but people risk it because of the potential for rich rewards.

Mutual funds: Mutual funds are a group holding made up of both stocks and bonds. As such, they hold medium risk. They are usually organized through your employer and maintained by a professional management company who invests the money for you.

Real estate: Real estate falls in the middle of the risk spectrum. It is rare that homes lose their value (though it is becoming more common), but it can take years before you see a return on your money.

Questions to consider yourself or ask a financial advisor include:

- What is your goal for investing (buying a house, college fund, retirement, etc.)?
- How much money can you part with?
- How long are you able to let your funds sit in an investment?
- How much of a risk are you willing to take?
- Do you prefer to be hands-on or have a professional handle your investments?
- Does your company offer a 401k, 403b, or other type of retirement savings plan?

ⓘ PREGNANCY FACT

Your baby's face continues to develop its character. If you could see your baby's face up close, you would see the arch of his eyebrows and the slightest bit of soft, downy hair. Likewise, his scalp continues to fill in with hair in a predetermined pattern. Also, around now, your baby's reflexes are becoming more frequent, and he may be startled by loud noises outside the womb. Thus, dogs barking, alarms, and your sneezes may send your baby into surprised somersaults!

If mom is involved in a car accident while pregnant, see the doctor right away or go to the emergency room. Even if the accident was minor and she feels fine, it is important to have a thorough exam. Even though baby is protected by the amniotic sac and fluid, there is a chance that the placenta can become dislodged. This can be very dangerous and could lead to preterm labor or even miscarriage. Thus, a thorough exam, including ultrasound, is necessary to make sure everything is as it should be.

The information in this section is cursory, but will help you get started. Ask family members, friends and coworkers who have investment portfolios how they built theirs. Personal experience is often the best indicator for what works and what does not. For example, find out if they use a brokerage firm, an online organization, or manage their own accounts.

Above all, take your time learning the lingo. Practice getting a feel for how the market works by picking a few stocks and following their progress before making a purchase. Any research you do now will make you feel more informed when you are ready to start investing.

COMMON QUESTIONS THAT DADS HAVE

In addition to being curious about how to provide for your family, you may have wondered about the following this month:

How big is my baby now? By the end of the fourth month, he will be about 6 inches long and weigh between 6 and 9 ounces. This means your partner's uterus has expanded a lot—the top hits the halfway point between her pubic bone and her belly button.

Is it safe for my partner to remain a vegetarian or vegan during pregnancy? Yes. As long as she eats the daily recommended requirements of each of the essential nutrients, her pregnancy will be just as healthy as pregnant omnivores. The major concern with non-meat eaters during pregnancy is that they consume enough protein, iron, and calcium. Luckily, all of these are abundant in various vegetables, legumes, and fortified grain products, such as bread and cereal.

Should my partner avoid taking acetaminophen while she's pregnant? Acetaminophen is considered safe to take during pregnancy. But if she takes it often for a persistent headache, let her doctor know—it could be a sign of preeclampsia.

I think my partner is gaining too much weight—should I tell her? In the interest of preserving the peace, the answer is "No way!" Telling a pregnant woman she is gaining too much weight is like poking a lion—ill-advised and dangerous. Your partner should be gaining about a pound a week, so by the end of this month she may have gained anywhere from 8 to 15 pounds. It really depends on her appetite and how sick she was during the first trimester. The best thing for you to do if you are truly concerned is to take over meal preparation and include lots of healthy snacks on your grocery list.

Will playing classical music to my child in the womb make him smarter? Researchers have tried for years to determine this, and the results are mixed. Some studies say yes, others say no. But all agree that playing music to baby in the womb is a way for dad to connect to his child. So feel free to conduct your own experiment

DID YOU KNOW?

The odds of miscarriage are low now, so many women choose to share the good news with friends, family, and coworkers at this point. For some, this can be the moment they've waited for all of their lives, while others find that telling people they are pregnant opens the door to unsolicited advice. Expect that you may be the recipient of pregnancy-related tales that run the gamut from the very touching to the absolutely tragic. Set limits with people who share only stories that increase your anxiety.

with Mozart, but keep a few things in mind. Studies show that amniotic fluid actually amplifies low-tones, such as bass. If played over 70 decibels, music can damage your baby's hearing. In addition to quiet music, reading and talking is an effective way to communicate with your unborn child. Some research indicates babies respond to the voices heard while in the womb.

How can I help my partner cope with back pain? Back pain is a common, persistent, and difficult symptom to manage during pregnancy. However, there are some definite steps you can take to help relieve some of mom's pain. Take on all lifting chores, including grocery shopping, laundry, moving furniture, as well as lifting older children or pets. There will times when mom must lift something heavy, but you should be doing the bulk of the work at this point. You can also encourage her to take warm baths at the end of the day, and massage her gently. You can also try rolling a sock full of uncooked rice that has been warmed in the microwave along the small of her back. For times when you are outside of the house, keep a soft pillow in the car for long outings like the movies or concerts. Your partner's tailbone gets sore from sitting on a hard surface, and she will appreciate the extra cushion. Also, purchase a body pillow for her to sleep with at night. Having a pillow or towel between her knees when she sleeps on her side will bring great relief. Finally, remind her to stretch and walk every day to keep her muscles elastic and strong.

HOW DAD CAN DEAL

Comedian Tim Allen once quipped, "My mom said the only reason men are alive is for lawn care and vehicle maintenance." While you are probably alive for a few other reasons, this is a good month to take on these more masculine home-improvement projects. They will keep your mind and body occupied, make you feel useful, and have mom tickled pink at your initiative.

Some projects to get started on this month include:
Replace batteries in existing smoke detectors or install new ones. Smoke alarms are your best chance for getting out of the house during a fire. But for the alarm to do its job it must be in working condition. Smoke detectors usually need fresh batteries every year. In addition to changing batteries in detectors, make sure to install one where your baby will sleep.

Put covers over exposed outlets. You would be surprised how many homes have exposed outlets or outlets with loose wires hanging out. Fix these before baby comes home, because lack of sleep and general busy-ness will prevent you from doing this later.

Start baby-proofing your home. Start collecting baby gates, plastic outlet plugs, foam runners for sharp corners, and other

✖ TIPS & ADVICE

For some men, pregnancy is a time of anxiety rather than joy—particularly if this is your first baby. Thanks to the age of online message boards, you do not have to go through pregnancy alone. If you find that you're up at 2 in the morning wishing for another father-to-be to talk to, try joining a chat room for men with pregnant partners. Online chat rooms and message boards are a great resource for tips on how to help mom manage symptoms, product suggestions, exercise tips, emotional support, and more.

items that help you make your home safe. If you are not sure what needs to be done, crawl around on the floor. Whatever you can see and reach, your child will be able to as well. Of course, it will be a while before she is able to get around, but it is never too early to start anticipating what ordinary household items might pose a threat to a child.

Paint the nursery. If you have the room for a nursery and want to paint the walls, now is a great time to do it. Feel free to get creative! Not all nurseries need to have ducks and blocks on the walls. You might draw a large tree with different colored birds in it, or an underwater fish scene. Or, if you're not much of an artist, colorful strips and swaths will do too. Just make sure to keep your partner out of the room while you paint, though, so she and the baby are not exposed to paint fumes.

Fasten furniture to the walls. Before you know it, your son or daughter will be cruising around the house. If a bookcase is not attached to the wall, there is a chance she could pull it down and get seriously injured. This project is also important for families who live in earthquake-prone areas. Take the time this month to secure furniture so you don't have to think about it later.

HOW DAD CAN HELP

Your role as support person and ambassador will come in very handy this month. As news spreads of your partner's pregnancy, everyone from the mail carrier to your mother will be coming forward with unsolicited pregnancy and childbirth advice. Handling these well-meaning but pesky folks is an important job that is just right for dad.

Your partner will really appreciate your help in situations where people want to share horror stories or tell her how to be pregnant. For some inexplicable reason, people think a pregnant woman wants to hear about miscarriages, stillbirths, labors that lasted 36 hours, and babies who succumbed to Sudden Infant Death Syndrome (SIDS). Of course, these often-exaggerated tales only increase her anxiety about childbirth, and thus, she should be shielded from them. In addition to stories that will terrify her, many people will feel compelled to tell her how eat, sleep, walk, and breathe while she is pregnant. This, too, will stress her out and may cause her to doubt herself. This is where you come in.

Whether you are present for these types of interactions or hear about them later, help mom out by doing the following:
- Publicly commend your wife for the great job she is doing with her pregnancy.
- Tell those who try to share terrible pregnancy outcomes that you appreciate their interest, but you are trying to stay positive and prefer not to hear such stories.

- Regularly reassure your partner that you and she are making the right decisions regarding management of her pregnancy.
- Remind your partner that some people get satisfaction from telling the worst story and assure her that neither of you needs that kind of person in your lives.
- Make it known to family members that you will not stand for criticism or scrutiny of the pregnancy.

Often, just taking a few simple but reassuring steps is enough to mitigate the droves of busy-bodies and naysayers. Most of all, she will really appreciate feeling that you are on her side.

HOW DAD CAN BE INVOLVED

The second trimester is time to lighten up and have some fun with your pregnant partner. So get creative about how to connect with her this month.

There are several ways dads can precipitate good times this month, such as:

- Have your photos taken in a booth that combines you and your partner's pictures to create a hideous version of your offspring. These booths can usually be found in arcades, amusement parks, or arcade restaurants like Dave & Buster's.
- Take pictures of your wife on the same day of each month and post them on the refrigerator.
- Offer to measure her belly—but only when she in the zone to enjoy it.
- Start a "The Year You Were Born," scrapbook for baby. Include clippings of important newspaper stories, photos of popular celebrities, movie listings, Billboard music charts, shocking weather news, stories about the president, airline tickets, receipts for special baby items, crazy meals your

Your partner may find herself on the receiving end of random belly-rubbers! These are friends or even strangers who act on the urge to touch mom's belly without asking. You can help out by developing a strategy for dealing with unwanted belly-rubbers. Help mom verbalize that she would rather not be touched. Say something like, "I'd rather you didn't touch her, please," while mom takes a step back. It may be awkward, but you will both be thankful later that you established boundaries now.

partner craved while pregnant, and photos of you and your partner, other kids, and pets.

- Share with your partner how you imagine feeling when you hold your son or daughter for the first time.
- Talk to your partner's belly, even if it feels silly.

DAD'S RESPONSIBILITIES

Most fathers-to-be find themselves pondering their own morality around this time. You might cringe when you remember that accident you almost got into or that time you stupidly walked to the edge of a sharp drop. Feeling your own vulnerability in the world is good because it helps you keep yourself safe and healthy.

This month, aim to reduce the number of unnecessary risks you take on the road every day:

- Drive slower
- Refrain from texting or talking on your cell phone
- Avoid the urge to eat and drive

✖ **TIPS & ADVICE**

Before you purchase big-ticket items, such as a crib, stroller, bassinet, high chair, or car seat, do your homework. All products are not created equal, and there are several agencies and organizations that test and rate products based on safety, cost, and durability. Some websites to check out include the U.S. Consumer Product Safety Commission (www.cpsc.gov) and Consumer Reports (www.consumerreports.org). It is a good idea to comparison shop and take your time before deciding on more expensive items.

- Quit smoking in the car
- Do not succumb to road rage
- Take care of necessary car repairs
- Park in well-lit areas
- Always wear your seat belt
- Purchase a roadside assistance plan

If you are already the model of safe driving, consider other areas in which you can protect yourself from harm. After all, it is more important than ever to reduce the number of unnecessary risks you take.

"A babe in the house is a well-spring of pleasure, a messenger of peace and love, a resting place for innocence on earth, a link between angels and men."
~ Martin Fraquhar Tupper

Lunar Month

Five

Second Trimester

Lunar Month five · · · · · · · · · 🦆

MONTHLY TO-DO LISTS

- ☐ Go with mom to her prenatal appointment
- ☐ Bring a video camera to the first ultrasound
- ☐ Try not to be jealous that mom can feel baby move and you cannot
- ☐ Slow down and wait up for your partner
- ☐ Take on additional chores and errands
- ☐ Expect your partner's sex drive to increase or decrease
- ☐ Start investigating daycare options
- ☐ Make a childcare budget
- ☐ Prevent mom from participating in sports such as scuba diving, sky diving, and gymnastics
- ☐ Encourage your partner to keep taking prenatal vitamins
- ☐ Discuss abnormal test results with your doctor or a genetic counselor

MY PERSONAL CHECKLIST:

- ☐ ....
- ☐ ....
- ☐ ....

MY HOPES FOR THIS MONTH:

....
....
....
....
....
....
....
....
....
....
....

What's Happening: Mom & Baby

Second Trimester

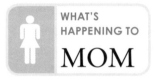

This month marks the halfway point in the pregnancy. This is an exciting milestone! One of the best experiences is to see your baby appear on the ultrasound for the first time. There is nothing quite like this experience. It is a moment of pure joy, even disbelief. Many parents can't believe that it is their baby they are watching wiggle, wave, turn, and swallow onscreen. Quite a few dads have been reduced to tears during this awesome and overwhelming moment.

The ultrasound is often the moment in pregnancy when the baby becomes a human presence to many parents. As a result, mom (and dad) may constantly touch her belly, frequently speak to baby, become obsessed with personal safety, and feel driven to start buying baby clothes, furniture, and toys. This drive to connect with the baby is kicked off by seeing her for the first time. It is then fueled by feeling her movements with regularity—an event known as quickening. Some time between 18 and 20 lunar weeks, mom will feel flutters that intensify. Most women find that babies are most active in the morning and at night, when mom is still. During the day, the baby is usually rocked to sleep by mom's activities. Mothers-to-be find these movements to be deeply comforting. Baby's

MOM'S Symptoms

- Darkening of face, breasts, and abdomen
- Back, joint and ligament pain
- Leg cramps
- Increased or decreased sex drive
- Hemorrhoids
- Varicose veins
- Shortness of breath
- Tires easily
- Headaches
- Constipation
- Nosebleeds and bleeding gums
- Heartburn
- Feet and ankle swelling
- Increased appetite
- Brittle nails
- Leaky breasts
- Forgetfulness
- Quickening

movements are a sign that she is alive and well, and keep mom company throughout the day. As mom's connection to her child deepens, so too will her desire to protect him from potentially harmful situations. As a result, mom may clamp down on whatever remains of your pre-pregnancy lifestyle. It may be hard for you to imagine more changes and cutbacks, since it probably feels like your lives have been altered so much already.

Your partner's raging hormones might have her contradicting herself a lot this month. She may enthusiastically agree to accompany you to a baseball game, for example, only to want to leave by the second or third inning because her back hurts, her feet and ankles are swollen, and she needs a nap. Muster as much flexibility and understanding as you can when your partner's disposition seems to come from left field. Even though it is annoying to constantly be changing the game plan, mom's body is the best judge of what is good for baby.

You can also expect mom to become increasingly forgetful as the months go on. This condition, dubbed "pregnancy brain," is maddening for moms and suspicious to dads. But despite its controversial legitimacy, forgetfulness affects the majority of pregnant women. Researchers are conflicted about the cause— some suggested culprits are hormones, excessive fatigue, and even temporary brain shrinkage. No matter its origin, absentmindedness is frustrating, annoying, and can even be dangerous. For example, mom may forget to turn off a burner on the stove or to lock the doors at night. Therefore, trail her at a discreet distance as she makes dinner or shuts the house up to take care of whatever she forgot to do.

Aside from having to leave baseball games early and making sure your wife doesn't burn the house down, the fifth month is a wonderful time for intimacy. Relief from nausea and vomiting may cause mom to feel sexy again. As a result, you can experience with more frequency the amazing pregnancy orgasm. It can take

DID YOU KNOW?

If mom hasn't already felt the baby moving, she will by the end of this month. For many women, having a baby doesn't feel real until they feel their wee one moving around with some regularity. Baby will sleep most of the day and may not move a lot during that time. Most women find that their babies are most active first thing in the morning and at night. Dad, however, must wait a little bit longer to feel baby moving—until baby is heavier and can punch and kick with some gusto.

mom anywhere from 2 seconds to 2 hours to climax, making for an interesting sex life. You may also notice that her breasts leak a bit when she is excited. This is normal and evidence that her breasts are filling up with milk to feed baby.

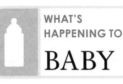

WHAT'S HAPPENING TO BABY

This month is baby's time to shine. Not only does he make his debut onscreen during the ultrasound, but he also moves so much that mom can feel him. The reason his movements are detectable at this point is because he has gained so much weight and length, his arms and legs actually make an impact when they hit the uterine walls. Indeed, by the end of the month he will be about 7½ inches long and may weigh between 9 and 15 ounces. His bones continue to harden, his hearing improves, he builds up more fat stores, and his skin becomes a little less transparent. What this means is that your baby is looking more and more like he will when he is born.

Adding to his human appearance is the hair he will sprout on his head and eyebrows this month. It is a very thin layer of fine hair that may not be visible on an ultrasound, but is there nonetheless. He is also developing a wax-like coating called vernix caseosa that protects his skin while in utero. Vernix is laid over lanugo, the hair that coats and protects your baby's body. The residual slippery substance that makes up vernix is also responsible for helping baby slide through the birth canal and out of the vagina. Beneath the vernix, baby's skin is developing its three layers—the epidermis, dermis, and subcutis. The third and deepest layer, the subcutis, is mostly fat. This is the one that helps the baby regulate his own body temperature after he is born. In addition to hair and skin development, baby's leg and inner ear bones continue to ossify. The hardening of the leg bones may be partly responsible for the fact that mom can feel baby's movements: it adds strength to his kicks. Inner ear development also contributes to his movement; when he hears new sounds, he may respond by moving. He may jump when startled by your car alarm or even tap along to music (not in time, of course).

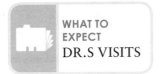

WHAT TO EXPECT
DR.S VISITS

Your partner will again have her urine tested and also get the Doppler monitor, which probably feel like old-hat by now. In addition, two additional tests will be discussed.

Amniocentesis: If last month's multiple marker test results were curious, your doctor probably recommended amniocentesis to clarify them. This test is performed in the doctor's office and is guided by ultrasound. Once the doctor picks a safe spot away from baby and the placenta, he will insert a long needle into the abdomen and pull about a tablespoon of amniotic fluid from the sac. This fluid will be analyzed for evidence of chromosomal and

✖ TIPS & ADVICE

If for any reason you do not feel comfortable and confident with your OB-GYN, switch doctors now and find someone you are both happier with. But assuming you are happy with your doctor, start talking with him about delivery day. Ask your doctor who will deliver your baby if he is not available. Your doctor will do his best to be there on delivery day, but there's always the chance that you will go into labor while he is on vacation. You can even ask to meet the back-up doctor, if it will help ease your mind.

genetic disorders—it will also be able to determine the sex of the baby. In some cases, amniocentesis is recommended even when the multiple marker screening was normal, such as if mom is 35 or older, if you have other children with chromosomal or genetic disorders, or you or your partner were born with birth defects. This test is optional, however, and so you and your partner must evaluate whether it is worth the risk—1 in 200 tests result in miscarriage.

Ultrasound or sonogram: An ultrasound is usually offered around 20 weeks (LMP). This optional diagnostic uses sound waves to create a picture as the doctor or technician moves a wand over your partner's abdomen. Ultrasound technology allows your partner's physician to determine whether mom is carrying a single child or multiples, track heartbeats per minute, measure baby's size, evaluate the health of the placenta, measure volume of amniotic fluid, and inspect baby's overall development.

What's Happening: Dad

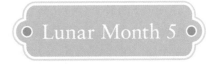

Lunar Month 5

Second Trimester

With each passing month, you get closer to really believing you are going to be a dad. And this fifth lunar month of pregnancy offers a mega-dose of this reality as you see your baby for the first time during an ultrasound.

WHAT DAD IS THINKING AND FEELING

Author Gabriel Garcia Marquez once said, "A man knows he is growing old because he begins to look like his father." This wise sentiment touches on the connection between father and son—not just the physical, but also the behavioral. Your outlook, decisions, and preferences all start to change as fatherhood approaches. And though you may not feel physically aged, you certainly cannot help but notice the choices you make are more responsible, self-sacrificing, and geared toward the unit rather than the individual. Your matured perspective is underscored this month by a very significant development—seeing an image of your baby for the first time on an ultrasound.

The effect of seeing your child is profound. It may result in you feeling like a puffed-up papa bear ready to protect your little cub. Or, you might be reduced to feeling like a helpless boy who is in way over his head. Both responses are normal and

> You can offer your partner support by making the same decisions and sacrifices that she is making for baby. For instance, if she is watching her calories carefully, it will not help her to see you eating pepperoni pizza while she eats a salad. You should try to eat what she eats and be sensitive to her cravings, restrictions, and aversions. And while it may be hard to turn down a beer or glass of wine, you can help make social events much more pleasant for your partner by abstaining from alcohol while she is pregnant.

eventually lead to the same sentiment of, "Wow, I am really going to be a father." The only difference between men who immediately feel ready and those who do not is that it takes longer for the latter to "age" in the way Marquez described. If you do not have the "Aha!" moment after the ultrasound, don't worry about it. Everyone comes to terms with the enormity of fatherhood in their own way and at their own pace.

This month, expect your partner to cry out, "Honey! I think I just felt the baby move!" You run to her, place your hands on her abdomen, and she says, "It stopped." You leave the room and 5 minutes later yells, "I feel it again!" Once again you place your hands on her abdomen, and she asks, "Do you feel it?! Isn't it amazing?!" Desperate to share in this moment, your hands slide all over mom's belly as she tries to direct you to the hot spot. Chances are you will not feel baby moving this time, or any of the next several times your wife calls out for you to come feel the action. Though your partner is lucky to experience quickening this month, it may be a while before you are able to feel baby's movements.

It is a disappointing moment for a dad who wants to be involved in every aspect of the pregnancy. You may even feel jealous as you see your partner's hands glued to her abdomen. A lot of men feel sidelined by a woman's early connection with the baby. But in a matter of weeks, you will have it too. Until then, ask your partner to describe what it feels like. Sharing, rather than begrudging these special moments will bring you closer to your partner, the pregnancy, and to your overall goal of maturing as a father-to-be.

THINGS DAD SHOULD KNOW

Another month brings more pregnancy-related vocabulary to learn. Pregnancy language can be confusing, and knowing the terms that make it up will prevent you from feeling in the dark.

Some of the following concepts are specific to the development of your baby while others have to do with mom and her symptoms:

Bradycardia: Heartbeat of less than 60 beats per minute

Candida infection: Infection caused by yeast buildup in mom's intestines or vagina—same as a yeast infection. Symptoms include itching and cottage cheese-like discharge.

Ectoderm: Germ layer tissue that forms the nervous system, epidermis, pituitary gland, and teeth

Endoderm: Germ layer tissue that forms baby's respiratory organs, bladder, vagina, digestive tract, and urethra

False labor: Braxton-Hicks contractions without the thinning or dilation of the cervix

DID YOU KNOW?

Around lunar week 18 (20 weeks LMP) you may have an ultrasound to determine whether you are having a boy or a girl. If you are having a girl, her uterus will have started to develop. If you are having a boy, his genitals will be plain as day on the ultrasound, unless your baby is camera-shy and facing the wrong way. Keep in mind that there is still a small percentage of error that occurs when a technician reads an ultrasound, so it is slightly possible (though unlikely) that you will have a girl even if you've been told "It's a boy!"

Fetal movement: The motions baby makes while in utero. These become an important indicator for evaluating his well-being.

Gravida: A pregnant woman

Hypertension: High blood pressure during pregnancy

Incontinence: Involuntary expulsion of urine from the bladder, most often as a result of pressure from the uterus

Kegel exercises: Intentional strengthening of vaginal muscles and bladder through concentrated flexing and releasing

Mesoderm: Germ layer of tissue that forms baby's muscles, connective tissue, and certain organs

Montgomery glands: Tiny bumps that rise around the areolas during pregnancy

Sciatica: Painful condition of the back that puts pressure on nerves and causes tingling or numbness in the feet and ankles

Spina Bifida: Birth defect of the spine that can be detected early with amniocentesis

Toxoplasmosis: An infectious disease caused by parasites found in infected cat feces or undercooked meat that can result in miscarriage or stillbirth

Wharton's jelly: Gelatin-like substance inside the umbilical cord that is abundant with stem cells

HELPFUL HINTS FOR DAD

Your baby's hearing is developed enough to start responding to sounds that travel into the womb. Take advantage of this development, dad, because this is your opportunity to connect with baby in your own special way. Besides, research shows that babies

✖ FOOD FOR THOUGHT

Start mom's mornings out right by serving her oatmeal for breakfast a few times a week. Oatmeal has been shown to lower cholesterol and is a heart-friendly food. There is also evidence it may reduce the odds of developing certain types of cancers. It contains several essential minerals and vitamins, including iron, fiber, protein, and complex carbohydrates. Because oatmeal slows digestion, it will make mom feel full longer and can help quell heartburn and nausea.

recognize sounds they heard in utero, such as mom and dad's voices, the family dog's bark, and theme songs of often-watched TV shows. One study conducted at the Foetal Behaviour Research Centre in Belfast, Northern Ireland discovered that babies born to mothers who watched a specific television show while pregnant became calm, quiet, and alert when the theme song to that show was played.

Though you cannot feel your baby move in response to your voice just yet, you can encourage recognition by making him familiar with your voice. Help "program" your voice in your baby's brain by laying next to your partner with your head propped up on a pillow next to her abdomen. Start talking and see what comes out! You may feel silly at first, but you will get used to having conversations with your baby while in utero. Ask your partner to let you to do this several times a week. Have her tell you when the baby responds to your voice. Eventually, you will be able to feel his movements on your own, but in the meantime this is an excellent way to bond with both mom and baby.

COMMON QUESTIONS THAT DADS HAVE

This month, the following might be on your mind:

Can my partner have a flu shot while pregnant? Flu shots are considered safe during pregnancy, so yes. If your partner was to get the flu with accompanying respiratory problems and a fever, her misery would be off the charts. In addition, high fevers can be dangerous to the fetus, so be safe and get the shot.

My partner keeps forgetting to take her prenatal vitamins. Is this a big deal? Prenatal vitamins are most valuable for their folic acid content, which is most important during the first 6 weeks or pregnancy. But the other vitamins and minerals in these

By now, mom is probably looking quite pregnant, as her uterus has grown to the point that it is level with her belly button. However, each woman "shows" in her own way, depending on her size and shape before becoming pregnant. Along these lines, you may have heard others claim all sorts of wisdom about your baby based on how high or low mom is carrying. However, there is no scientific evidence that supports a correlation between the shape of a woman's belly and the gender of your baby.

supplements can only help baby's development, so it is wise to take them throughout the course of pregnancy. Encourage your partner to take her vitamins by taking yours with her. Say something like, "Let's take our multivitamins at the same time—otherwise I'll forget."

My partner is still suffering from morning sickness. Is this normal? It is normal, but rare: About 1 in 7 women experience pregnancy symptoms beyond their 20th week. If she is unable to keep any food or water down, tell her doctor. She may be dehydrated and require medical attention.

What sports or exercises should my partner avoid? Most activities are fine as long as your partner stays hydrated and respects her body's limits. However, certain sports are considered dangerous during pregnancy because of the potential for injury or miscarriage. These include biking, skiing, sky diving, SCUBA diving, horseback riding, and gymnastics. Never let your partner participate in any of these while pregnant.

> If you are thinking of skipping childbirth education classes, think again. Classes are often held in the hospital where mom will give birth and end with a tour of the labor and delivery floor. This alone is worth the cost, as it helps demystify the environment in which you will have your baby. Also, these classes are full of important information. You will meet other expectant parents and be able to share your experiences with them. Check with your insurance company as many offer free or inexpensive classes.

Is it wrong that I want to have sex with my partner constantly? Of course not! It is perfectly normal to become hyper-attracted to your partner. After all, she is more curvy and voluptuous, which is very sexy to most men. She may or may not be able to match your stamina, so it is important not to push your needs on her. If you find your desires do not match up, suggest other means of sexual expression besides intercourse.

HOW DAD CAN DEAL

It is possible that some of the tests mom had this month or last came back with troubling results. Learning that everything might not be normal with your baby is disappointing, difficult, even terrifying. Before getting too upset over abnormal test results, learn as much as you can about the test and the margin of error included. For example, receiving a "screen positive" result for neural tube defects after the multiple marker screening does not mean you should panic. It does mean that your partner should consider further testing, such as having amniocentesis. It also means you should speak at length to a genetic counselor or your doctor about how to interpret the results. These experts can explain whether the test simply indicates the need for more testing, or if it reveals an actual problem with baby's development.

Furthermore, there is a chance that the test reported a false positive, which means the test was wrong and your baby is fine. For this reason you and your partner may consider more accurate diagnostics. However, because such tests are very invasive, many couples choose to stop here and hope for the best. It depends on how far your family is willing to go to "know," and what you are prepared to do in the event your worst fears are confirmed.

Finally, if the worst is confirmed, discuss with your doctor options for terminating the pregnancy. This is difficult for any couple who has invested so much time, energy, and emotion in the pregnancy. But some birth defects are so severe that giving birth is more traumatic than terminating the pregnancy, even at this late a stage. Should you find yourself in this tragic situation, seek professional counseling immediately.

HOW DAD CAN HELP

Since most American households require two incomes to function, it is likely that your partner will return to work within 6 months of giving birth. Unless you plan to be a stay-at-home-dad, you will need reliable, trustworthy, and affordable daycare. Though it may seem too early to plan for childcare, nothing could be further from the truth. Once your son or daughter is born, you and your partner will be adjusting to parenthood, working on very little sleep, and have little time to do anything but care for your newborn. Besides, many popular daycare centers are booked months, even years in advance and require parents to sign up on a waiting list. You'll also need time to establish your childcare budget, interview potential providers, and decide what type of daycare is right for your family's needs. Taking on the responsibility for researching daycare options this month will be a big help.

Before you dive in to interviews and create a budget, break the childcare issue down into digestible components. Doing so gives you the confidence to make informed decisions.

The first step is to understand the different types of daycare arrangements:

Grandparents: For most couples, having a grandparent watch their baby is ideal. You both know and trust your parents, it is usually both financially liberating and worry-free. Grandparents as nannies are not necessarily an entirely cost-free situation, however. Some grandparents may feel taken advantage of or may feel too free to cross lines established by you and your partner. Since they are not hired help they may be less inclined to follow your instructions or parenting styles and feel that they "know best."

In-home nanny: Hiring an in-home nanny that shows up on time and goes home at the end of the day is every mother's dream and every father's financial nightmare. This is generally reserved for higher-income families. If you can afford it, it is worth the cost. Nannies give 100 percent of their attention to your child. In addition, they are often educated in childhood development. In many cases, they are backed by reputable agencies who conduct thorough background checks, which saves you a lot of time and effort.

Nanny share: Nanny-share situations are popular these days and a great solution for cost-conscious parents who want the benefits of having a nanny. Putting this together is as simple as going in with other families who all use the same nanny and splitting the cost. Of course, the fee is higher because there are more children

DID YOU KNOW?

Fetal heart development goes through many stages. In each of these stages, your baby's heart will resemble that of a particular animal—from a fish to a snake and, finally, that of a human. Once your baby is born, his heart will be roughly the same size as his fist. As he grows, so will his heart—keeping pace with the size of his fist throughout his life. Heart size can often indicate heart health—for example, an enlarged heart often indicates cardiac distress and a small heart points to developmental issues.

to watch, but most nannies offer a reduced rate when caring for more than one child. There are some challenges that accompany this arrangement. Every family must agree where the nanny will care for the children—tricky when everyone wants their kid at their own house. However, your child will still get individualized attention for less than it would cost to have your own nanny. And, your child will be socialized from an early age, which is important to his development.

Live-in au pair: An au pair is usually a young, unmarried woman from another country who lives with a host family. She is viewed as a member of the family who does childcare and some housework for room, board, and monetary compensation. Rates and conditions of employment depend on the arrangements made with the agency that represents her.

✖ TIPS & ADVICE

Be sure you and your partner make time for intimacy. Keep in mind it will be much more difficult to make time for just the two of you when there is a newborn to care for. So, each morning or evening, turn off the television, don't answer the phone, and cuddle up with mom. The physical closeness will do wonders for both of your stress levels, and if it leads to sex, that's great! Unless you've been ordered by your doctor to avoid penetration or orgasm, sex is perfectly safe—and beneficial—for you and your partner.

Out-of-home professional daycare facility: Daycare facilities are usually the least expensive childcare option. These facilities are able to keep costs down by caring for many children at the same time. Private facilities or religious organizations are the exception, as these can cost more than $4,000 a month. But smaller community daycare centers usually have reasonable rates with long waiting lists. When using this type of facility, make sure they are licensed and that they adhere to the mandated adult-to-child ratio set by your city or state.

Daycare provided at a personal residence: Daycare run in personal residences is becoming increasingly common. These small businesses are usually run by mothers who are home with their own children and are looking to earn an income. Many are licensed, but some are not. You must use your judgment whether this matters to you. For example, if your wife's best friend is running an in-home daycare, you may not care that she is not licensed. The same operation run by a stranger, on the other hand, may make you nervous. If you can find an acceptable person, this is usually an affordable option with flexibility that other daycare options do not provide.

HOW DAD CAN BE INVOLVED

Since there is little for you to do with the pregnancy this month, you can be involved in other ways, such as researching daycare options. A huge part of this job is conducting interviews with providers. Of course, deciding which type of daycare is right for your family is the first step. But even after you narrow down your preferences for in-home versus out-of-home care, your selection may ultimately be decided by information gathered during your investigation of specific providers.

Once you select the type of care, set up tours of facilities and interviews. Offer to include your partner in these, but if she trusts your judgment, feel free to run with the process.

When visiting a daycare center or in-home facility, pay attention to the following details:

- The adult-to-child ratio
- Education level of staff
- How many children under age 2 are enrolled
- How many infants under 6 months are enrolled
- Cleanliness
- Condition and safety of toys and furniture
- Whether the center is baby-proofed
- Whether there is a safe, fenced-in outdoor play area with shade
- The condition of the kitchen
- Whether the children seem happy, agitated, or stressed
- How many cribs there are for naps
- Whether there are cats or dogs

If you are satisfied by what you see, dig deeper. Conduct interviews with the facility. You'll want to talk to the manager of the operation and with anyone who will have direct contact with your child.

The following is a list of questions to ask either an in-home or out-of-home provider:

- How long have you been a daycare provider?
- What brought you into the childcare business?
- What experience do you have with infants?
- Do you hit or spank children?
- Is anyone ever on-site that does not work here, such as a husband, boyfriend, or friend?
- Will you agree to a background check?
- How many employees do you have and how long have they worked for you?
- Do you conduct background checks on your employees?
- Are you comfortable with unannounced visits by parents?
- Have you ever been convicted of a crime?
- Are you certified in infant CPR/first aid?
- Are you a licensed daycare provider?
- What activities do kids do while here?
- Is your facility equipped with smoke detectors and fire exits?
- Do you have a valid driver's license?
- Do you have a plan for evacuation in case of fire?
- Do you provide meals?
- Are you prepared to watch a child with allergies or special needs?

Next, talk to other parents who use the daycare. Ask them why they use this provider. Also, drop by the facility a few times, unannounced, and just observe. If you feel satisfied, begin a background check.

ⓘ **PREGNANCY FACTS**

Ancient Egyptians believed that children were a blessing and so families generally had between 4 and 15 children. The Egyptians used many salves and plant remedies to aid the mother in her delivery. The Ancient Egyptians believed that pregnancy lasted between 271 and 294 days. When it was time to give birth, the mother squatted, sat, or kneeled on a birthing seat. Often, a pot of hot water was placed below her, because it was thought that the steam would make her delivery easier.

DAD'S RESPONSIBILITIES

Families spend 25 percent or more of their annual income on childcare. Daycare costs anywhere between $100 and $1,000 per week. This month, your responsibility is to find a daycare option you can afford and begin financially planning for it. Seek out providers within your price range or slightly higher, as your income can be expected to rise slightly each year. Avoid thinking that more expensive means better. In some cases this is true, but reasonably priced childcare can be just as developmentally healthy for your child as a private preschool. The most important thing is to trust your provider to take excellent care of your child in your absence.

It will help you to know that you can claim a federal tax credit of up to 35 percent of eligible childcare-related costs. You need your provider's tax ID or social security number to file for the credit. Also, find out if your company offers childcare reimbursement. Sometimes you can set aside pre-tax money from each paycheck into a special childcare account.

+ HEALTH CONCERNS

Vacationing at altitudes of 7,000 feet or above can be dangerous for your baby. This is because it will take awhile for mom's already-taxed respiratory and circulatory system to adjust to the lower oxygen levels. In fact, she may not adjust fast enough to supply necessary oxygen to baby, which can cause fetal distress. If you must go to a high-elevation destination, make sure to ascend no more than 2,000 feet per day. Also, book your accommodations below 6,500 feet so you are sleeping in a more oxygen-rich environment.

Another option is to set aside pre-tax income in a Flexible Spending Account (FSA). The money in this account is not taxed and reduces the amount of your income that is taxed. For example, if you earn $40,000 a year and set aside $4,000 in an FSA, you will only be taxed on $36,000 of your earnings. However, there are limitations on some of these scenarios—you can't use both the federal childcare tax credit and the dependent-care account, for example—so research which option benefits you the most.

"Pregnancy is a process that invites you to surrender to the unseen force behind all life."
~ Judy Ford

Lunar Month

Six

Second Trimester

MONTHLY TO-DO LISTS

- ☐ Attend prenatal appointments with mom if you can
- ☐ Sign up for childbirth classes
- ☐ Enroll in an infant CPR/first aid class
- ☐ Enroll in other newborn classes, such as dogs-and-babies class
- ☐ Take over all heavy lifting
- ☐ Offer to do most of the driving
- ☐ Help your partner get up from lying or sitting down to reduce round ligament pain
- ☐ Assuage mom's fears about labor and delivery
- ☐ Try out new sexual positions, such as letting your partner be on top
- ☐ Go with mom to register for baby shower gifts if she is having a shower

MY PERSONAL CHECKLIST:

- ☐ ....
- ☐ ....
- ☐ ....

MY HOPES FOR THIS MONTH:

....

....

....

....

....

....

....

....

....

What's Happening: Mom & Baby

Lunar Month 6

Second Trimester

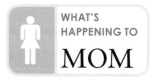

WHAT'S HAPPENING TO MOM

Lunar month 6 is the last month in the second trimester and also the start of the second half of pregnancy. It is considered a transitional time of pregnancy because although she is probably starting to feel anxious about labor and delivery, your partner's moods have likely stabilized. Indeed, around the 22nd week of pregnancy, the amount of progesterone and estrogen produced by mom's body are about equal. However, the levels of both hormones are 10 times greater than in a non-pregnant woman. High hormone levels are necessary to support the many body changes mom experiences this month. For example, they are helping your partner's breasts fill with milk. As a result, her breasts continue to enlarge and her nipples may protrude through her clothing. She may also leak a thin yellow liquid called colostrum. The milk production going on within mom's mammary glands may cause her breasts to weigh up to 1½ pounds more than before she was pregnant! The good news is that your partner should not have breast pain or tenderness at this point, unless she has a clogged milk duct. This will feel like a little lump and be marked by red skin and tenderness at the site. They can be treated with warm compresses and by wearing soft-cup bras.

MOM'S Symptoms

- Varicose veins
- Constipation
- Headaches
- Dizziness
- Congestion
- Nosebleeds
- Bleeding gums
- Leg cramps
- Heartburn
- Increased appetite
- Hemorrhoids
- Round ligament pain
- Vaginal discharge
- Leaky breasts
- Increased fetal movement
- Back pain
- Itchiness
- Swelling of ankles and feet
- Numb or tingling sensation in wrist and fingers
- Stretch marks
- Forgetfulness

This month, mom's uterus will have stretched from the size of a pear (in lunar month 1) to about the size of a basketball. The top of the fundus is about 2½ inches above her belly button, so she is definitely looking pregnant. All of this stretching can cause sharp, severe, stabbing pains called round ligament pain. These are most intense when getting up from a laying or seated position. Encourage your partner to get up slowly—it will reduce the intensity of these spasms.

In addition to dealing with round ligament pain, mom will also be surprised by sporadic contractions this month. Called Braxton-Hicks contractions, or false labor, this tightening and releasing of the uterus is normal and does not mean she is going into preterm labor. Braxton-Hicks contractions act as the body's practice for when real labor begins. They come at irregular intervals and should be painless—unlike mom's lower back pain, which will become the focus of her misery this month. Unfortunately, there is little to be done about increasing back pain at this stage. The pain is coming from movement in her spine, which curves backward to make room for her ever-expanding belly and breasts. In addition, the hormone relaxin is causing her joints and ligaments to loosen to make it easier for baby to exit the womb during childbirth. With looser joints and ligaments, mom's lower back is forced to work harder to stabilize her body. As a result she is feeling muscle tension, chronic back pain, and even sciatica (pinched nerves that cause numbness and tingling in her feet).

You may notice your partner has started walking funny this month. Women often develop the "pregnancy waddle" as they adjust to their new center of gravity. You will recognize the waddle by its signature outward-pointing feet. Try not to make too much fun of your waddling partner—she may be on edge this month as her anxiety about getting this baby out of her mounts.

It is very common for women to freak out this month. There is something about the changes that occur in the sixth month that causes pregnant women's attention to switch from pregnancy to labor and delivery. As the newness of pregnancy falls away, her

ⓘ PREGNANCY FACT

It is likely that your partner is feeling as if she will be pregnant forever. You can help by doing things together that have nothing to do with pregnancy. If you haven't already taken a weekend getaway, now is the time to plan one, dad! Another great way to make mom feel pretty and special is by arranging a spa day and then going out for a nice dinner for two. Remember to take advantage of this "just the two of us" time because soon it will be "and baby makes three."

thoughts turn to fearing childbirth. She may seem jumpy, edgy, or snap and cry more than usual. She may even beg you to make her not go through with it. Rest assured that though mom will be nervous from now until delivery day, she will not be at this level of anxiety the entire time.

With emotions running high, hormones leveling off, and mom's increased voluptuousness, you may notice that your partner wants to have sex more than in previous weeks and months. This is a positive development and one to act on if you can. A lot of men report feeling intimidated by their partner's large size and fear squashing or even "denting" the baby. Letting your partner get on top can help you feel more comfortable with having sex at this stage in the pregnancy. Your partner is likely to have a few contractions after she orgasms—as long as her pregnancy is progressing normally, these are normal, safe, and nothing to worry about.

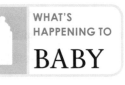

WHAT'S HAPPENING TO BABY

At the beginning of this month your baby is still very thin, and not quite the cherub you picture when you imagine your child. But within a few weeks he will start to pack on ounces as he becomes able to swallow and digest tiny amounts of sugar present in the amniotic fluid. This is sweet timing, because his tongue is also starting to form taste buds. Though he still has much weight to gain, by the end of the sixth month, your baby will be up to 15 inches long and weigh between 1½ and 2 pounds, dramatically increasing his chances of surviving preterm delivery. While you want your child to stay in the womb for as long as possible to maximize his development, it is important for a baby to be able to survive an early delivery should one occur. Babies born at this weight in the sixth month have about a 50 percent chance of survival.

DID YOU KNOW?

Now that you are nearing the end of the trimester, consider how to commemorate this special time in your lives. One excellent way is to photograph mom's belly at the beginning of each new month. Another great idea is to keep a pregnancy journal that details things like how you both felt, when you first felt the baby kick, and what it meant to hear the heartbeat for the first time. If you haven't already started doing these this, it is not too late to start. Pick up the camera and your journal, and get busy.

Your child's chance of survival is also enhanced by the fact that this month his bone marrow starts working in conjunction with his liver and spleen to produce blood cells. His lungs start producing a substance called surfactant, which his lungs need to inflate. And though he receives oxygen through the placenta, he is taking practice breaths by inhaling and exhaling amniotic fluid. This is excellent practice for life "on the outside." Despite these advances, lung development is not complete until baby reaches full term.

WHAT TO EXPECT DR.S VISITS

Another month brings another checkup. You can expect the usual routine of urine sample, physical, and hearing baby's heartbeat amplified through the Doppler.

There are also three new tests that may be offered:
Glucose challenge test (GCT): Your partner will be asked to drink a sugar solution that contains 50 grams of glucose. She will

✖ TIPS & ADVICE

> To deal with the forgetfulness typical of this stage of pregnancy, get mom a daily organizer. Or, better yet, hang a large dry-erase calendar on the inside of your front door so that she can see a daily task list as she leaves the house. This all may seem very strange but "pregnancy brain" forces you and your partner to become quite resourceful to stay on top of everything.

sit for an hour and then give a blood sample. The results of this test indicate her risk for developing gestational diabetes. If your partner's blood-sugar level is high she will take a follow-up test or her doctor may start treating her for gestational diabetes.

Glucose tolerance test (GTT): GTT is the follow-up to the GCT. For 3 days prior to it, mom will eat 150 grams of carbohydrates daily and then fast for 8 hours before the test (schedule it for the morning). Your partner will give a blood sample once an hour for 3 hours. The results will clearly indicate whether mom has developed gestational diabetes.

Fetoscopy: If your child is at high-risk for severe birth defects, your partner may be encouraged to have a fetoscopy. The doctor will make a small incision in her abdomen and insert a fetoscope, guided by ultrasound. This instrument can take pictures as well as collect samples of baby's blood, tissue, and umbilical cord. Fetoscopy can determine whether the baby will suffer from inherited diseases or physical birth defects.

What's Happening: Dad

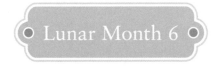

Lunar Month 6

Second Trimester

As the second trimester comes to a close, it is common for dads to feel both suffocated and excited at the same time. Like mom, you may be anxious about labor and delivery and be concerned you won't get everything done before baby arrives.

WHAT DAD IS THINKING AND FEELING

As discussions increasingly turn toward what needs to happen before baby is born, it is possible that the connection you worked so hard to make with your partner has begun to feel like a chore. Indeed, around this time, many men start feeling trapped, controlled, and even consumed by the urge to flee. If you entertain such thoughts, it doesn't mean you are a bad person or that you'll be a terrible father. The sixth month of pregnancy brings up a series of complex thoughts and emotions that may require some introspection to sort through.

Of course, getting enough quiet time to yourself these days may be difficult since your partner needs your help and support more than ever. Her increasing dependence on you is one factor that makes you feel stifled and trapped. Another is your loss of identity—while you used to pass your time tinkering around in the garage, playing tennis, or noodling on guitar, much of your time is now dedicated

+ HEALTH CONCERNS

From now until the end of pregnancy, heartburn will be mom's companion. Though it is safe to take Tums or Mylanta (with your doctor's approval), taking steps to prevent or avoid heartburn is a better course of action. Help her avoid spicy, fatty, or acidic foods. She should wait at least two hours after eating before lying down. If heartburn is particularly bad, she can try eating a small portion of plain oatmeal made with reduced-fat milk. This can be soothing and soak up some of those excess acids.

to making mom's life easier and preparing for baby's arrival. This shift in how your time is spent may not have been a big deal at first. But once the sixth month hits your partner's constant requests may have you feeling caged. Examples include asking you to pick up something on your way home from work, skip your workout, turn down social invitations, reach this, carry that, read this, and bring me that. The specifics will vary from couple to couple, but the basic situation is the same—your partner has something for you to do every minute of every day, and thus your time is no longer your own.

In some ways, this loss of independence is good practice for after baby is born. The reality is, once you go back to work and your partner is left alone with a newborn, she is likely to tighten the reins even more. But before you pack a bag and head for the hills, give some thought to your partner's perspective. Try to imagine how trapped mom must feel—she cannot escape her physical ties to baby. You, however, are physically free from the symptoms and risks of pregnancy, labor, and delivery.

Moreover, an unfortunate truth about pregnancy is that you and your partner will rarely be on the same page at the same time. This can exacerbate feelings of alienation and frustration, not to mention encourages desperate—and ill-timed—attempts to force a connection. When you sense your partner trying to force something on you, you probably resent it and retreat. But when you pull away, it enhances mom's insecurities about your love and attraction for her—causing her to try to reel you in by controlling your time. Nobody wins in this situation.

Thus, your job this month is to put an end to this cycle by communicating your frustration with mom. Find a gentle way to explain that you feel suffocated. Assume she feels the same way and talk about it as a team. Establish some boundaries. Claim at least one day a week, or an hour every few days, that is your time to do whatever you want—even if this means doing nothing more than laying on the couch, eating potato chips and surfing the

🔍 DID YOU KNOW?

If mom is carrying multiples, she is at higher risk for preterm labor. Therefore, it is very important that you know when to call your doctor. Some symptoms, such as Braxton-Hicks contractions are not cause for concern. However, if she experiences any of the following, call your doctor right away: pelvic pressure or fullness, more than four contractions in an hour, cramping that does not go away, ruptured amniotic sac, discolored vaginal discharge, or bleeding. If she has more than one of these at the same time, head to the hospital.

The sixth month is a great time to purchase a few books about caring for a newborn. There are several reputable guides that will come in handy when it is 3 a.m. and you are wondering if your baby's poop should be that color. Starting your library now will cut down on last-minute runs to the bookstore will also help you to feel more prepared when you bring your bundle of joy home. You should either go to the bookstore while mom rests, register for the books, or order them online.

Internet. Let her know that allowing you to have this time entirely to yourself keeps you from being frustrated. It also makes it more likely for you to help out during the rest of the week without being asked. Your partner is likely to see that she has more to gain by giving you a bit of space.

THINGS DAD SHOULD KNOW

The following is a list of terms to add to your pregnancy vocabulary. Some may not come up during your partner's pregnancy. But in case they do, you will be prepared to understand what is being discussed.

Anomaly: A physical abnormality in relation to baby's development

Antibody: Substance produced by the immune system to attack bacteria or infection

Cerclage: Surgery to close the opening in an incompetent cervix to prevent preterm labor

Edema: Swelling as a result of the extra fluids present in the body during gestation

Endocrine: Glands that produce hormones

Fibroid tumors: Benign growths within the uterus

HELLP Syndrome: Stands for Hemolysis, Elevated Liver Function, Low Platelets. This condition is a severe form of preeclampsia that causes the destruction of red blood cells. The only cure is to deliver baby to save mom.

Premature: A baby who is born before 37 weeks

PUBS: Stands for Percutaneous Umbilical Blood Sampling. Invasive procedure where a needle is inserted into the amniotic sac and the umbilical cord to test for fetal abnormalities.

Vanishing twin syndrome: When one of two fetuses disappears in the womb, leaving just one baby

HELPFUL HINTS FOR DAD

If you and your partner have decided to take childbirth education classes, now is the time to sign up for them. They fill up quickly and the classes you prefer may not be available before your baby is due. Besides, most classes run between 6 and 12 weeks long, and instructors recommend couples finish their classes by the 38th week. Take the lead on discussing with your partner the types of classes available and then start calling around.

Begin with your medical insurance company. Many offer classes for free or for a nominal fee. If you do not have insurance or if yours does not offer childbirth classes, check the phone book or do an Internet search.

There are many kinds of classes out there, and you'll want to decide which are best suited to you and your partner.

Lamaze: The most popular method in the U.S., the Lamaze philosophy focuses on natural birthing while controlling pain through quick-patterned breathing. Moms like it because they feel in control of their labor and dads like it because they get to play the significant role of mom's coach. Lamaze classes teach mom how to breathe by panting to control pain. Dad's job is to help his partner concentrate on a focal point. Mom is encouraged to come up with a list of labor tools to have on hand, such as a stress ball, essential oils, and relaxing music. Dads are taught how to massage mom during labor, how to communicate with nurses and doctors, and how to keep mom as comfortable as possible. The Lamaze philosophy is opened-minded about pain medication and respects the need for Cesarean, but most of the focus is directed toward giving birth naturally. Classes run between 6 and 8 weeks and classes are 2½ hours long.

The Bradley Method (TBM): The Bradley Method also supports natural labor and delivery. In fact, about 94 percent of TBM moms give birth without use of pain medication. TBM differs from Lamaze in that it focuses on good nutrition and exercise during pregnancy. Another difference is that while Lamaze emphasizes panting and shallow breathing, The Bradley Method teaches women to take deep, slow breaths. Also, TBM encourages women to concentrate on the sensations going on inside her body instead of on a focal point in the room. Similar to Lamaze, TBM dads are taught how to coach mom during labor and delivery through

A good recommendation for mom is to attend a breast-feeding support group while she is still pregnant. Spending time with new mothers who recently went through labor and delivery can be a great educational experience. New moms are eager to tell their stories and to help other moms learn from their experiences. Asking a few of the mothers to share their stories, and what they wished they had known or asked or done, can give you and your partner invaluable tools heading into your own baby's birth.

encouragement and physical contact. TBM classes run 12 weeks long and also focus on postpartum issues such as breast-feeding.

International Childbirth Education Association (ICEA) Classes: ICEA classes are a great choice for parents who do not feel married to a particular discipline. This is because ICEA instructors cover several methods and encourage students to work with whatever is most comfortable for them. Classes cover natural childbirth, pain medications, Cesarean section delivery, breast-feeding, and bonding with baby.

Hypnobirth®: Hypnobirth® is a natural childbirth method that teaches mom to use self-hypnosis, visualization, and deep relaxation techniques. The founding principle is that childbirth does not have to be painful if mom is sufficiently prepared and relaxed. In a Hypnobirth® setting, dad acts as a guide for mom, taking her into deep states of relaxation, giving hypnosis cues, and reminding her to use visualization. Though emphasis is placed on giving birth naturally, Hypnobirth® instructors touch upon use of

> ### ⓘ PREGNANCY FACTS
>
> If you are the first among your group of friends to be expecting a baby, be prepared for some major changes in your friendships. Though you are all are well-meaning and want to try to keep things as they are, things will be different. Your needs and priorities will become different enough that you may find yourself seeing your friends much less than before you were a dad-to-be. This can be a difficult transition, but those who are committed to your friendship will stick around and become part of your baby's life.

pain medication during an emergency Cesarean. Classes run for 5 weeks for 2½ hours or for 4 weeks at 3 hours.

Birthing from Within®: Birthing from Within® classes are taught by "mentors" who encourage parents to be accepting of their childbirth circumstances. This includes going in without having a desired outcome—such as a vaginal delivery. Classes focus on controlling pain through self-hypnosis, meditation, mindfulness, and medication if needed. It is a holistic approach to childbirth that emphasizes learning through dialogue with other parents in the class. Classes are offered in weekend power sessions, four 3-hour Saturdays, or spread out over 6 weeks.

There are benefits to all childbirth education methods and, on some level, they all cover the same basic structure of labor and delivery. Where they differ is in their approach for coping with pain. Since she'll be the one grappling with the pain issue, the decision for which class to take should ultimately be up to your partner. But make it known which kind of class you prefer. Some dads want to be on the receiving end when baby is born, while others are happy to station themselves near mom's shoulders. Some want to take an active role in coaching their partner and some want to let her take the reins on the experience. At the end of the day, the most important tool both you and your partner can bring to the childbirth experience is an open mind and the willingness to change it when true labor starts.

COMMON QUESTIONS THAT DADS HAVE

Perhaps you are contemplating the following this month:

My partner wants to dye her hair, but I heard it's dangerous to the baby. Who is right? There is no evidence that the occasional application of hair dye will harm a fetus. However, if your partner happens to be a cosmetologist who dyes hair 40 hours a week, she might want to hang up her rubber gloves until after she has the baby. Only that level of exposure to fumes could potentially affect the baby's development. But if your partner

---

🔍 DID YOU KNOW?

You may be surprised to learn that you already have control over determining how your baby's tastes for food will develop. Studies have shown that babies are influenced by the flavors they taste while in utero. So, if you want to raise a child who will eat his veggies, be sure mom ingests plenty of them while pregnant and also when she is nursing. Similarly, babies exposed to high doses of sugar while in utero or when breast-feeding may be slower to accept foods that are not sweet.

✖ FOOD FOR THOUGHT

A great way to have a healthy and easy home-cooked meal is to make a cream of vegetable soup. Sauté one small yellow onion and a clove of diced garlic in a tablespoon of olive oil. Add a nutrient-rich vegetable—broccoli, asparagus, or potatoes are great selections—then sauté until coated with the garlic/onion mixture. Add one carton of vegetable broth, bring to a boil then let simmer until vegetables are soft. Finally, puree the mixture in a blender and return to the pot. Add ½ cup of low-fat milk, stir, and serve!

just wants to touch up her roots or have a beauty day, she is in the clear—just make sure she is in a well-ventilated area.

When should my partner stop working? When to take maternity leave is decided by mom and her doctor. Of course, you can throw your two cents in, but if you want your partner to work up until labor starts to keep the money flowing, you are fighting an uphill—and potentially dangerous—battle. On the contrary, if you ask your partner to stop working before she is ready she may resent the request. The best way to approach this subject to ask your partner what her plan is and then be prepared for it to change as the pregnancy progresses.

When will I be able to feel my baby kick? There is no one answer to this question—it depends on how big your baby is, how thick or thin your partner is, and if you are lucky with your timing. You probably have a few more weeks to go before you will be able to feel your baby kick or punch.

Is it wrong that I don't feel like going to all of the prenatal appointments? Definitely not. Odds are, your partner doesn't feel like going once a month either! If the appointments conflict with your work schedule or cut into other errands you have to run, aim for going to every other appointment, or just to the "big" ones—when an ultrasound is scheduled or you expect to receive test results, for example.

We like to travel. When do we to have stop flying? You still have some time before your partner is advised to stop flying, so get trips out of the way now while you can. Most doctors suggest that women who are having a normal pregnancy avoid flying after 36 weeks. And in most cases, the airlines take the decision out of your hands anyway by refusing to allow women who are within 2 to 3 weeks of their due dates to fly, in case they go into labor.

Should I tell my partner I don't want her mother to stay with us after the baby is born? Yes, but be careful how you say it. This is a delicate matter that must be handled with diplomacy and tact. Suggest that her mother come after you return to work so you have the initial few weeks to bond as a family. Remind her that her mother's help is likely to be most helpful when you are gone during the days, anyway. Focus on what you want from those first few days and weeks instead of why you do not want her mother there.

HOW DAD CAN DEAL

Continue preparing yourself for fatherhood by enrolling in any number of baby preparation classes. These are specialty courses that differ from childbirth classes in that they focus on how to handle various situations after you bring your son or daughter home.

If you do not already have a life insurance policy, start shopping around for one. You will need coverage for both you and your partner. You will first want to figure out what it costs to run your household annually. Be sure to include the added cost of having a new baby. It is advisable to purchase 6 to 10 times your yearly salary in coverage. Also, it is customary to have your partner be the recipient of the benefits, so that if something happens to one of you the other will have enough money to take care of the family.

The following list of classes teach valuable lessons for how to care for and keep baby safe—as well as for how to introduce and include older children and pets into your baby's life.

Infant CPR/First aid: This class is a must for all new parents—even for those who are certified in adult CPR. Knowing how to perform CPR and first aid on an infant is crucial to avoid injuring his tiny body and breaking his ribs. In this 4- or 5-hour class you will learn to recognize when there is an emergency, how to make sure the scene for rescue is safe for you and baby, how to save a baby who is choking, what to do during a cardiac emergency or when a baby is not breathing, and when to call 911 and what to say. The American Red Cross, The American Heart Association, and other organizations offer in-person and DVD-instructed courses.

Getting Ready for Baby: There are several different names for this type of class, but the sentiment is the same for all of them. Instructors use a doll to teach parents how to change a diaper, swaddle or wrap, breast-feed, and hold a newborn. Basic care is also discussed, such as how many wet diapers to expect, how to bathe your newborn, umbilical cord stump care, circumcision, baby's first visit to the doctor, his first shots, first poop, and other key matters. Classes run about 4 weeks for 2 hours each.

Introducing Pets and Babies: Parents who are pet owners should take this excellent class run by the Humane Society. Instructors have first-hand experience with the subject matter and are passionate about integrating your baby as one of the pack. This one-day course teaches parents when to keep pets and babies separate, when it is OK to introduce them, how to introduce them, how to keep your pet from becoming jealous, and why it is important for your pet to have a safe, quiet retreat that is off-limits to baby. In addition, instructors give practical advice for how to walk with a stroller and a leashed dog and how to avoid forcing your dog to love your baby.

New Baby for Siblings: Many hospitals have 2-hour classes for older children that explain what it means that a new baby is on the way. Siblings are given a tour of the hospital and made to feel that they are an important member of the family—and of the baby's birth. Children are given "jobs" for when mom is in labor and delivery, either at home or at the hospital. These classes reduce feelings of jealousy or alienation in older children.

HOW DAD CAN HELP

Nowadays, it is customary for friends or family to throw a baby shower for a pregnant friend. It is even becoming acceptable for dad and his friends to be invited. The shower usually occurs a month before the baby is born, but it can start being planned around now. To make gift-giving easier for guests, most couples establish a registry—similar to a wedding—at a few stores. Setting up the registry is easy but time-consuming and requires a bit of research and a few trips to the store. Offer to go with mom to register for items you hope to receive before baby arrives.

There are a few points to consider when establishing a gift registry:

Consider how the pregnancy is progressing: The bridal shower is a leftover tradition from World War II when communities of women would rally to help an expectant mother in need. The tradition has morphed into an event not everyone is comfortable with. Many cultures do not have parties until after a baby is born—some do not even give the baby a name for quite some time after the birth because of the risk of infant mortality. Therefore, if you and your partner are nervous about having a shower—don't have one. Especially if she has a high-risk pregnancy or is expected to have an especially difficult labor and delivery. In these instances, you may want to plan a party for some time after the baby is born and mom's health is stabilized.

Register for what you need: When parents are in a store with the magical register wand, their urge is to scan giant teddy bears and baby-sized recliners. Within the first few weeks you will curse your decision and wish you had registered for diapers and wipes instead of the cute but useless fluffy infant robe and slipper set. Make sure to cast a more realistic eye on the registry process so you end up with things you will really need, like blankets, clothes, and bottles.

Don't bank on getting everything you need from the registry: There is nothing wrong with hoping a benevolent family member will purchase the $400 stroller-and-car-seat combo you registered for. But be realistic about how many big-ticket items you include on your registry. The bulk of the registry should be made up of items that cost between $10 and $50. When people can

ⓘ PREGNANCY FACTS

You may have noticed that mom's belly button has popped out and now shows through her clothes. This is a normal part of pregnancy that occurs as the uterus pushes upward. Mom may not mind this, or she may find it annoying to see her belly button through her shirts and dresses. If so, there are products on the market that she can buy to place over her belly button to tape it down. And for those moms-to-be whose belly buttons don't pop out at all—don't worry, this is also completely normal.

comfortably afford the options, you are likely to get more gifts. A more realistic strategy is to budget for major purchases such as cribs, changing tables, gliders, car seats, and strollers and then register for less-expensive items.

HOW DAD CAN BE INVOLVED

One way for dad to be involved this month is to look into banking or donating your baby's cord blood after birth. This process is a way to harvest and store valuable stem cells that are in the umbilical cord. These stem cells may be used later in the event someone in your family develops a serious illness. However, there is a lot to consider before a final decision is made. Collecting cord blood is not yet a routine hospital procedure and requires advanced planning and a contract with a private agency. Storing your baby's cord blood can cost between $1,000 and $2,000, plus an annual fee of $100 to $500 per year, plus additional costs required by the individual companies who provide the service. There is no definitive evidence of how long cord blood stays "good," and the stems cells harvested from the umbilical cord can only be used on children or babies. If you decide not to bank your child's cord blood, consider donating it to a nonprofit agency, such as the American Red Cross or the National Donor Marrow Program.

DAD'S RESPONSIBILITIES

Your responsibility this month is to quell mom's anxieties by getting family affairs in order. This includes keeping up with your list of home-improvement projects, making a budget, filing paperwork, and planning for childcare. As you start getting your life in order, mom will be able to relax a little.

"Childbirth is more admirable than conquest, more amazing than self-defense, and as courageous as either one."
~ Gloria Steinem

Lunar Month

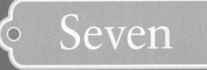

Seven

Third Trimester

Lunar Month seven . . . .

MONTHLY TO-DO LISTS

- [ ] Continue to go to childbirth classes
- [ ] Be on the lookout for signs of preterm labor
- [ ] Consider hiring a doula
- [ ] Expect a decrease in your partner's sex drive
- [ ] Be creative to maintain intimacy with your partner
- [ ] Know when to call the doctor
- [ ] Make sure mom doesn't try to lose any weight
- [ ] Help your partner start counting baby's kicks
- [ ] Reassure your partner that the heart palpitations and fluttering she feels are not signs of a heart attack
- [ ] Use your knowledge of gestational diabetes and preeclampsia to keep mom calm, should these conditions affect her

MY PERSONAL CHECKLIST:

- [ ] ....
- [ ] ....
- [ ] ....

MY HOPES FOR THIS MONTH:

....

....

....

....

....

....

....

....

....

What's Happening: Mom & Baby

Third Trimester

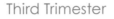

WHAT'S HAPPENING TO MOM

MOM'S Symptoms

- Shortness of breath
- Hot flashes and fatigue
- Varicose veins
- Constipation
- Belly button popping out
- Headaches and dizziness
- Congestion
- Nosebleeds
- Bleeding gums
- Leg cramps and back pain

The seventh month is an exciting milestone. It marks the beginning of the third and final trimester. However, it is also a rough time for mom as many symptoms reappear or occur for the first time, taking a huge toll on her body. Aches, pains, weight gain, and extra fluids all contribute to mom's growing impatience with her pregnancy. As a result, she may become more irritable, fatigued, and ready for pregnancy to be over. It is important for dad to anticipate this sudden downturn in his partner's disposition.

Many of the symptoms that emerge this month are a result of your partner's expanding uterus. Remember that at the beginning of pregnancy,

MOM'S
Symptoms

- **Heartburn and nausea**
- **Increased appetite**
- **Hemorrhoids**
- **Round ligament pain**
- **Vaginal discharge**
- **Leaky breasts**
- **Increased fetal movement**
- **Itchiness of belly skin**
- **Swelling of ankles and feet**
- **Numbness or tingling**
- **Stretch marks**
- **Forgetfulness and insomnia**

her uterus was about the size of pear and sat several inches below her belly button. By this point in the pregnancy, mom's uterus has stretched to just a few inches below her breasts and is about as big as a soccer ball! This causes her to take quick, shallow breaths even though her lung capacity has increased significantly. In fact, in order to accommodate the extra room needed for mom's lungs to fully inflate, her rib cage will expand up to 3 inches by the time baby is born.

Adding to your partner's upper body discomfort is the development of an occasional irregular heartbeat. It is normal, yet unsettling, for mom to experience flutters and skipped or extra heartbeats. Her heart may pound during activities such as walking up stairs, exercising, and even after eating. It feels this way because her heart is working twice as hard as it was before she became pregnant. Knowing this, however, does not make it easier to bear when it is happening. In fact, your partner may have occasional panic attacks—not only is her heart beating faster than normal, but she also cannot take deep breaths to bring it under control. Your job during these episodes is to keep mom calm until the flutters pass. Mention it to her doctor if she needs extra reassurance or if the problem seems abnormal.

A pounding heart and shallow breathing are not mom's only problems this month. Her huge uterus is putting a lot of pressure on her stomach, bladder, and intestines, crowding them out to make room for baby. The pressure on her stomach will probably discourage her from eating large meals. She will also experience intense heartburn as the hormone relaxin has slackened her esophagus and made her digestive system slow to process food. These factors may make her as nauseous as she was in the first trimester. In addition to digestive issues, pressure on mom's intestines and bladder can increase instances of constipation and make it impossible for her to completely empty her bladder. This can make her susceptible to urinary tract infections (UTI). Signs of a UTI include fever, pain during urination, frequent urination, and peeing dark-colored urine. If your partner suspects she has a UTI, encourage her to get treatment—otherwise it can lead to preterm labor.

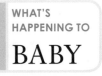
WHAT'S HAPPENING TO BABY

At the beginning of the seventh month, your baby has approximately 97 days left before she is born. She has developed to the point that if born today, she would have an 85 percent chance of survival (with special care from the NICU). One reason for baby's boosted chance of survival is that her lungs now produce enough surfactant that her air sacs inflate enough to breathe air. Of course, she still has a lot of developing left to do before her birth day comes. But most parents find it comforting to know that with each passing day their child gets closer to being able to live outside of the womb.

With all of the fetal activity lately, it may seem as if baby is trying to climb her way out of the uterus and into the world. The seventh month is when baby's activity levels become more intense and regular. By the middle of this month, you should be able to feel your baby's kicks when she is most active—usually first thing in the morning and late at night. The increase in activity is due, in part, to her size—by month's end she will be up to 16 inches long and weigh between 2 and 2½ pounds. In addition, her hands and feet are functional. Now that she has them, she wants to use them! Mom may be able to feel her "walk" around the walls of her uterus, tug on the umbilical cord, and push, punch, and kick throughout the day.

Your baby is also exploring her small world in other ways. For example, she can open and close her eyes, yawn, swallow, and hear and recognize mom's voice—maybe dad's, too. All of these activities stimulate her and encourage movement. Although she has established a regular sleeping pattern by now, she only sleeps for about 30 minutes before waking up. Like with a newborn, sleep is an important part of a fetus's development, so make sure there is lots of quiet time for your partner—and baby—to rest.

Sleep is important for giving fat a chance to build up under her skin—over the next several weeks, in fact, one of her main developmental goals is to put on weight. Between now and when she is born she will gain another 4½ to 6 pounds. At this moment,

✖ FOOD FOR THOUGHT

Beginning this month, mom should consume an additional 300 to 350 calories each day to keep up with baby's nutritional demands. Make sure that these are high-quality calories, and keep in mind it is possible to get these calories (and then some!) from just a few bites of a fast-food cheeseburger. Instead, mom should add calories to her diet by eating healthy snacks in between meals, such as a sliced apple with 2 tablespoons of peanut butter—this nutritious snack equals just 310 calories.

DID YOU KNOW?

Unfortunately, symptoms from the first trimester may surface and resurface for mom this month. The following will likely appear or increase this month: whitish vaginal discharge, sensitive and bleeding gums, congestion and nosebleeds, cramping in her calves, heartburn, constipation, hemorrhoids, varicose veins, headaches, insomnia, and backaches. The good news is you should both know some effective tips and tricks for relieving symptoms by now. It will also help to remind her that she is in the home-stretch of pregnancy.

she is tall, skinny, wrinkly, and red with thickening eyebrows and hair. But as she fills out, she will start to look more like the newborn you imagine.

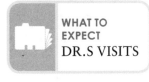

WHAT TO EXPECT
DR.S VISITS

In addition to the usual tests, this month your partner's doctor will ask about the frequency of baby's movements and may even ask her to start tracking them. At this stage in pregnancy, he may be concerned about the development of preeclampsia or early labor.

Your partner will also be asked to undergo the following tests:

Abdominal exam: Your partner's doctor will measure the height of mom's uterus from her pelvic bone to the top of her uterus. Mom's due date may be adjusted based on this measurement. In addition, the doctor may be able to feel baby's position—whether she is facing head-down or in a breech (upright) position.

Usually, if you and mom notice spotting or very light bleeding after sex or a medical examination, it is not cause for concern. It can be attributed to slight injury to the sensitive cervix. However, you should always alert your doctor if mom experiences any bleeding in the third trimester. In some cases it indicates something very serious is going on, such as the result of a low-lying placenta, separation of the placenta, a tear in the uterine lining, or premature labor.

Hematocrit/hemoglobin: This blood test is identical to the one your partner had in the first trimester to test for anemia. It is necessary to test for anemia again due to the increase in blood production.

Rh antibody screening: If your partner is Rh negative, the Rh antibody screening from the first trimester will be repeated. She will then be given a shot with Rh immunoglobin around week 28 and again after baby is born.

Ultrasound or sonogram: An ultrasound is usually offered one more time during the third trimester—sometimes more often if mom has gestational diabetes or there are other complications. This diagnostic test uses sound waves to create a picture as the doctor or technician moves a wand over your partner's abdomen. Ultrasound technology allows your partner's physician to see baby's heartbeat and track the beats per minute, measure the baby's size and age, evaluate the health of the placenta, measure the volume of amniotic fluid, inspect the baby's physical development, and determine the baby's sex with a reasonable amount of accuracy.

What's Happening: Dad

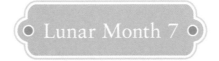

Lunar Month 7

Third Trimester

The beginning of the third trimester may kick your nerves into overdrive as the reality of fatherhood speeds toward you. Rather than being a sign that you are not ready, it is more a signal that you have begun to truly accept the weight of your new responsibilities. As 19th-century British philosopher Bertrand Russell once wrote, "One of the symptoms of an approaching nervous breakdown is the belief that one's work is terribly important." In this spirit, devote this month to turning a serious eye toward your child's impending birth.

WHAT DAD IS THINKING AND FEELING

The onset of the third trimester can make dad feel like the pregnancy is progressing at warp speed. This month allows the light at the end of the tunnel—baby's birth—to shine a little too brightly. This month, talk has likely turned from pregnancy to labor and delivery. You begin childbirth preparation classes, which are also focused on life after pregnancy. No longer cushioned between the first and third trimesters, you may feel anxious about your role as support person and like time is running out to sufficiently prepare before baby's arrival.

Ironically, childbirth preparation classes are often a source of both comfort and anxiety. Classes are comforting because they

+ HEALTH CONCERNS

There are some causes of premature labor that you can control. First, mom should never be exposed to secondhand smoke. Alcohol and drugs (including over the counter and herbal), standing for many hours in a row, regularly lifting heavy loads, infection of the gums, and being either severely under- or overweight can similarly increase her risk of going into early labor. Hopefully, you have given up many of these behaviors a long time ago, and now is more critical than ever to do so.

educate parents about what to expect during labor and delivery. They give dad a defined role with specific, yet flexible instructions and prepare mom to manage her pain during labor and delivery. However, both you and your partner may become overwhelmed by the wealth of detailed information you are given. Many men have trouble with the visual presentation of the information, in particular. Watching childbirth videos that show vaginal and Cesarean deliveries—close-ups included—is often disturbing for men, leaving them feeling queasy and unsure about their ability to handle themselves on the birth day.

These scenes may send you running from class—but don't give up. Your fear, even disgust, with the birthing process is completely normal, especially for men. Talk to some of the other men after class to find out what they think. If no one fesses up, be brave and the first to admit you are nervous and even repulsed by what you've seen. Like dominoes, it often only takes one man to admit he is freaked out to get others to talk. Once you start discussing your fears with others you will realize how common they are.

At this point, it can be helpful to sort your feelings into two categories: What I Can Do Something About, and What I Have No Control Over. Once you accept there are many aspects of the pregnancy, labor, and delivery that you have no control over, you can stop obsessing over them. Instead, focus on what you can control—like getting ready for baby's arrival. You still have at least 10 weeks left to prepare. When your imagination runs wild with visions of bloody show and giant needles, direct it toward one of the many ongoing projects you have started. This is an excellent way to stay centered and block out negative images that will distract you from supporting your partner.

THINGS DAD SHOULD KNOW

There is a lot to be nervous about this month—particularly mom going into early labor. If your partner is having a normal, healthy pregnancy, the chances of preterm labor are minimal. According

DID YOU KNOW?

There are many causes of preterm labor you have no control over. Those who suffer from a hormonal imbalance, incompetent cervix, premature cervical effacement, placenta previa, or an irritable uterus are all at higher risk for going into preterm labor. Unfortunately, these conditions or physical reactions won't be determined until mom is actually pregnant, so they aren't preventable. The best thing you can do for mom is to educate yourself about premature labor. Know the signs, so if you enter it, you can act quickly.

> You and mom may be thinking about when she will return to work after the baby is born. Put off making your final decision until she is at home with your newborn for a few weeks. Many mothers who decided they would not return to work find they do not enjoy the confines of staying at home. Still, other women find they have no interest in returning to their jobs once they get a chance to be a mom. Maternity leave protects employment, so it is better to see what it is like to be home with baby before making this critical life choice.

to the National Institutes of Health, just 12.7 percent of babies are born prematurely. You should also know that there are steps that can be taken to delay birth. This is important, because every day baby spends inside the womb is another day for her to become more able to survive on the "outside." Finally, you should thoroughly acquaint yourself with preterm labor and premature baby issues should your child be one of the 1 in 8 babies who are born before 37 weeks.

Preterm labor does not always equal a premature birth. It is possible in some cases to stop labor from progressing—but time is of the essence.

If your partner exhibits the following symptoms, call her doctor immediately:

- Contractions that come every 10 minutes or less
- Bleeding or a gush of fluid from the vagina
- Lower backache
- Pressure from baby on lower abdomen

- Cramps with or without diarrhea
- Nausea and vomiting

Should preterm labor start, your partner will look to you for reassurance. It is important for you to be strong and put on a brave face. You will probably be terrified, but don't tell your partner. She will undoubtedly be more scared than you. Listen carefully to the doctor's instructions and relay them to your partner slowly and clearly.

The doctor may suggest that your partner:
- Lay on her left side for an hour
- Drink 2 to 3 glasses of water or juice
- Meet him at his office or the hospital for an exam

Many times, the symptoms will pass, and in this case mom should stay home from work, rest, and monitor her condition. If symptoms persist or return, get your partner in to see her doctor. Depending on how far along mom is, her doctor may suggest medical intervention to stop or delay labor long enough for baby's lungs to mature further—even just 2 more days in the womb can make a significant difference.

To buy additional time, the doctor may try to delay delivery by using the following methods:

Bed rest: Mom may be laid up either at home or in the hospital. If she is in the hospital, her bed may be tilted so that her uterus is raised above her head. This prevents the baby from putting pressure on her cervix. Relieving gravity's pressure can be an effective way to delay early childbirth.

Home Uterine Activity Monitoring (HUAM): If mom is deemed high-risk for going into early labor, she may be outfitted with a HUAM to wear twice a day for an hour each time. The device is worn as a belt around her abdomen. It records the number and intensity of uterine contractions and transmits this information to her doctor for evaluation. HUAM is traditionally used for women carrying multiples, with health complications, or with a history of preterm labor.

Medications: Drugs called tocolytics are given either orally or intravenously to stop contractions. Medications in the tocolytic family include calcium channel blockers, terbutaline, ritodrine, magnesium sulfate, indomethacin, ketorolac and sulindac. They all have side effects ranging from mild to severe for both mom and baby. Your partner's doctor will decide which is the best option based on mom's health. Slowing down labor this way may buy between 2 and 7 days before baby is born. During this time, mom is injected with a corticosteroid to help baby's lungs mature more quickly. In addition, corticosteroids reduce the chances of bleeding in baby's brain and the development of necrotizing enterocolitis—a very serious bowel disease. Mom is also given antibiotics to prevent infections in both her and baby. Since premature newborns do not have fully developed immune systems, they are prone to many types of infections both during delivery and after birth.

Even if all of these methods are employed, there is a chance your partner could give birth to your baby before 37 weeks. Women who are younger than 19, older than 35, or who are carrying multiple fetuses are at higher risk for preterm delivery, though it technically can happen to anyone. The good news is, with the excellent care that neonatal intensive care units (NICU) provide, 90 percent of premature babies who weigh just slightly less than 2 pounds survive.

This is a good month for you to double as a forklift, as your partner will probably need some help getting up off the couch or out of the bathtub. The added strain of these motions on her abdomen, hips, and lower back can add to her overall achiness. Also, you should absolve mom of all heavy-lifting duties, even just carrying groceries and laundry. Carrying these will not harm mom or your baby, but relief from these duties will give your partner's back a much-needed break.

HELPFUL HINTS FOR DAD

By the end of this month, dad may feel overwhelmed by his looming responsibilities associated with labor and delivery. If you fall into this category—and even if you don't—consider hiring a doula. Doula means "woman who serves" in ancient Greek. This is fitting, because a doula's job truly is to serve mom during labor, delivery, and, in some cases, the early postpartum days.

A licensed doula is present during labor and delivery and can offer:

- On-call service 24/7 for up to 3 weeks before mom's due date
- Meetings with mom and dad between one and three times (or more, to be arranged with doula based on a fee) before baby is born to help mom prepare
- The help of a knowledgeable liaison to act as a go-between with medical staff and mom and dad
- Help keeping mom calm, relaxed, and informed
- Coping techniques for dad during the birth

+ HEALTH CONCERNS

If you are expecting triplets, you may be extra nervous about how your babies will enter the world. Though it is true that most women who are pregnant with triplets end up delivering at least one baby through Cesarean section, it is possible to experience vaginal delivery with at least one of the babies. This, of course, requires that mom and babies are in good health. But if the baby who is closest to the birth canal is head down, odds are good that this baby, at least, will be delivered vaginally.

- Training to handle the emotional needs of mom during labor and delivery
- Help with creating and sticking to a birth plan
- Help communicating with medical staff to gather as much information as mom needs to make informed decisions
- Help understanding how important the birth experience is for mom and preserving positive memories

Based on various surveys and clinical studies, the benefits of having a licensed doula present at labor and delivery include:

- Mom and dad feel more confident going into the experience
- Shorter labor
- Doula will often return calls sooner than the doctor's office
- Fewer complications
- More support for both mom and dad
- Less tension between mom and dad during labor
- Relieves dad from engaging in tasks he is not comfortable with
- Frees dad to interface with family and friends
- Fewer requests for pain medication

- Reduced need for labor-inducing drugs, such as Pitocin
- Can help explain birth-related medical terminology (although not a replacement for medical staff)
- Reduced need for Cesarean delivery
- Reduced need for delivery tools, such as forceps and vacuum extractor
- Mothers rate the overall birth experience more positively than those who do not use doulas

Hiring a licensed doula offers the following postpartum services and benefits:

- Support for the transition from hospital to home with newborn. This is important for new parents who have a hard time adjusting to lack of sleep and the demands of an infant. Families who use doulas for postpartum support have an easier time integrating their baby into their lives and have lower instances of abuse.
- Breast-feeding assistance. Mothers who have help from a doula have a higher success rate with breast-feeding because they are less likely to become frustrated and give up.
- Moms who use doulas are less likely to suffer from postpartum depression. The emotional and logistical support from a doula often boosts mom's confidence in her ability to care for a newborn.

If you and your partner decide to hire a doula you can expect to pay between $300 and $1,000, though the average cost is $500. Starting your search now will give you time to interview a few candidates and weigh their fee with the services they provide. There are several ways to find experienced doulas, such as by visiting any of the following agencies' websites: Doulas of North America (www.dona.org), the Association of Labor Assistants and Childbirth Educators (ALACE) (www.alace.org), Birth Works

> ### 🔍 DID YOU KNOW?
>
> The neonatal intensive care unit (NICU) is a section of the maternity ward where babies born with special medical needs reside until they are healthy enough to go home with their parents. Pediatricians developed the NICU in the 1950s to provide babies with protection from infections in a temperature-controlled incubator where they receive respiratory support from specialized machines. Babies in the NICU are allowed few visitors and even parents are required to wear protective gear when spending time with their baby.

(www.birthworks.org), Childbirth and Postpartum Professional Association (CAPPA) (www.cappa.net), and the International Childbirth Education Association (ICEA) (www.icea.org).

All doulas offer the same basic services. Therefore, the most important aspect of these meetings is to gauge the chemistry between mom and doula. Feeling comfortable with the person is the most important factor when selecting a doula.

COMMON QUESTIONS THAT DADS HAVE

The following questions might be lingering this month:
Will a doula eclipse my role as my partner's support person? No. A doula's main job is to tend to mom's emotional and physical comfort during labor and delivery. She can do this without stepping on your toes. Doulas are trained to facilitate communication between mom and dad, but if there is some job—such as cutting the umbilical cord—that you want to do, tell your

partner and the doula. Both will respect and encourage your desire
to participate.

**Should I be worried that our baby is not facing head down
yet?** No. There is still plenty of time for her to shift her position
before mom goes into labor. Sometime before labor begins, she will
drop down in to mom's pelvis, hopefully head first. When a baby
is feet- or rear end-down, she is considered breech. If baby stays
in the breech position, the doctor may try to turn her or suggest
mom have a Cesarean delivery. But at this point, you have nothing
to worry about.

**Is it appropriate for me to go out on the town with the
guys before my baby is born?** Definitely. Get out and enjoy the
world while you still can! Just don't go out so often that you leave
your partner home feeling abandoned, stuck, and lonely. Since
she cannot indulge in a last hurrah, she may not be sympathetic to
headaches, hangovers, or overspending, so don't go overboard.

✖ TIPS & ADVICE

Now that your partner's prenatal visits are scheduled
every two weeks, you are hopefully becoming close to
your doctor's staff. Making sure the nurses and front desk
people remember you will make visits more pleasant and
productive. Their memory of you can lead to increased
attention, such as call-backs over small concerns.
Maintaining good relationships with your doctor's staff,
and treating them with respect and patience, makes it more
likely that they will return your call sooner.

Is it true that I can expect to spend more than $7,000 on supplies for my baby in the first year? Yes. Costs of setting up the nursery with a crib, changing table, rocker, and other furniture—plus necessities such as a car seat, stroller, diapers, clothes, and toiletries easily exceed $7,000. You can cut costs by shopping around, using coupons, and watching for sales on big-ticket items. It is not recommended that parents purchase secondhand car seats or cribs due to potential safety concerns, but other secondhand or passed-down items are perfectly fine.

Will my partner ever want to have sex as often as she used to again? Yes. It may take awhile for her to get back to wanting it regularly, but her sex drive will return. Be prepared to deal with a continued dry spell after baby is born, because exhaustion, breast-feeding, and constant physical contact with the baby are likely to delay her sex drive's return for up to a year.

HOW DAD CAN DEAL

It is likely that your partner's sex drive has taken yet another nosedive this month, leaving you frustrated and unsatisfied much of the time. You might share some of mom's concerns about having intercourse—such as fear of hurting the baby or inducing labor. But chances are, you are game for at least some form of sexual expression that your partner does not share. So, what can you do to relieve tension and meet your needs?

This is a tricky time to turn to things like masturbation and pornography. Despite the fact that you are very attracted to your partner, if she finds pornography around the house or on your computer, she will take it incredibly personally. Remember that she is feeling fat, hungry and all-around unattractive many days. She is already worried that you won't find her as sexy and beautiful now

> **ⓘ PREGNANCY FACTS**
>
> Epidurals are the most popular childbirth pain relievers used for both vaginal and Cesarean births. The popularity stems from an epidural's ability to keep mom awake during delivery, since it causes only localized numbness. This means that mom is numb from her chest to her feet and does not feel any pain associated with the delivery of her baby. If you choose to have an epidural, be prepared for mom to have some side effects as it wears off, such as itching and shivering.

that she is pregnant. You don't want to exacerbate these feelings of insecurity, especially while hormones are surging and emotions are unpredictable. Be open and honest with your partner about your desires, but be careful. She is likely to misinterpret some actions as rejection of her.

No matter what outlet you use, continue to find ways to seduce your wife into intimacy. Think sparkling apple juice (instead of champagne), a nice dinner, a foot massage, and her favorite movie. Or bring her home flowers or a small gift to remind her how amazing you think she is. And, never stop telling her she is beautiful and sexy. Making a play for intimacy helps her feel attractive, boosts her self-confidence, and fosters a sex life under difficult circumstances. This will prove an asset in the coming months, because, unfortunately, new parents have to work on having the time and energy for sex for up to the first year after baby is born. So, lay the groundwork now for open discussions on how to maintain a sex life that is both realistic and satisfying to avoid either of you feeling isolated or undesired.

+ HEALTH CONCERNS

Some women choose to forego drugs during labor and delivery in favor of alternative methods of pain relief. Options include hypnosis, which causes mom to become extremely relaxed, but focused. Another popular method for pain control is acupuncture. Needles are placed in key areas on the skin by a professional. Both methods are more readily available in birthing centers than in hospitals— though it is possible to bring a practitioner in with you with clearance from your doctor.

HOW DAD CAN HELP

The best way you can help out this month is to understand pregnancy complications that may arise and learn ways to keep mom calm through them.

Your partner may face any number of surprise developments this month that will frighten her:
Gestational diabetes (GD): Being handed a gestational diabetes diagnosis can send mom reeling. Help keep her calm by understanding some facts about GD. GD is temporary and will go away once baby and the placenta are delivered. The majority of women with GD are able to manage their condition through diet and exercise alone. For women who need more help, medication deemed safe during pregnancy is available. Women with GD are closely monitored by their OB-GYN, a dietician, and a specially trained GD nurse.

Preeclampsia: A preeclampsia diagnosis at this stage is alarming, but you can help mom's blood pressure from skyrocketing by assuring her that she and baby will be fine with proper treatment. Depending on the severity of the condition your partner may need to go on bed rest or be admitted to the hospital for observation. She may also need to get medication intravenously to control her blood pressure. This means she will have to take maternity leave and, quite literally, stay in bed either at home or in the hospital until baby is born. Since there is no cure for this condition except for delivery of the baby, if her status becomes critical, her doctor may have to deliver the baby early. Therefore, it is very important that mom follow her doctor's instructions to the letter.

Vaginal bleeding: Bleeding may be serious and a sign of placental abruption, placenta previa, or hemorrhage. Other reasons for bleeding include injury to the cervix after intercourse or internal exam, internal bleeding after a car accident, or from an unknown cause. Bleeding should be reported to the doctor immediately.

HOW DAD CAN BE INVOLVED

If you and your partner have decided to hire a doula, make it your responsibility to set up interviews. Be present and ask questions. Get a feel for how your partner responds to the doula being interviewed, make note, and remind your partner of her reaction to each of the candidates. Also, encourage her not to "settle" for someone she did not make a connection with, and assure her there is plenty of time to find the right doula for the job. Make sure to ask if the doula is available around the due date, if she is licensed, with which organization or company she trained, how many births she has participated in, if you can contact other clients for references, and any other burning questions you have.

DAD'S RESPONSIBILITIES

Your responsibility this month is to thoroughly understand the signs and symptoms of preterm labor and know when to call the doctor. Moms usually come in two varieties: one that calls the doctor for every little thing, and one that never calls the doctor for fear of being a nuisance. Help your partner call when appropriate by understanding which situations warrant a phone call and which do not.

"Birth is the sudden opening of a window through which you look out upon a stupendous project."
~ William Dixon

Lunar Month

Eight

Third Trimester

Lunar Month eight · · · · · · · · ·

MONTHLY TO-DO LISTS

- ☐ Continue to attend prenatal appointments
- ☐ Continue to attend childbirth preparation classes
- ☐ Help your partner create a birth plan
- ☐ Learn some creative pro-pregnancy sexual positions
- ☐ Pack bags and be ready to go to the hospital in the event your baby comes early
- ☐ Remind mom to drink 8 to 10 glasses of water a day to reduce swelling
- ☐ Educate yourself about labor and delivery
- ☐ Find a male relative or friend to talk to about feelings of inadequacy or worry over becoming a father

MY PERSONAL CHECKLIST:

- ☐ ....
- ☐ ....
- ☐ ....

MY HOPES FOR THIS MONTH:

....

....

....

....

....

....

....

....

....

....

....

....

What's Happening: Mom & Baby

Lunar Month 8

Third Trimester

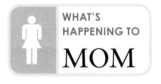

WHAT'S HAPPENING TO MOM

The eighth month of pregnancy puts mom right in the middle of the third trimester. This sets the stage for a conflicted emotional state—your partner is anxious to be done with the pregnancy, yet also feels sad it is almost over.

She may experience mood swings as a result of these feelings, but most of the time she will be focused on her physical state. By this time, her uterus is nearly the size of a watermelon. It is pushing up, down, and out in every direction. The weight of it may be pressing on mom's sciatic nerves, causing intense back pain along with numbness or tingling in her toes. This very uncomfortable condition is temporary, and should go away once the baby shifts position or after delivery. In the meantime, she will have trouble getting comfortable, particularly when sitting for a long time.

In addition to sciatica, mom's protruding belly, heavy breasts, and loosening joints will cause both lower and moderate to severe upper back pain this month. Lifting, bending, and staying in one position for too long will exacerbate regular back pain, as well as sciatica, so help her out in these areas.

MOM'S
Symptoms

- Back pain
- Leg cramps
- Heartburn and gas
- Indigestion and nausea
- Constipation
- Incontinence
- Headaches
- Dizziness
- Fatigue
- Congestion
- Bleeding gums or nose bleeds
- Achy abdomen
- Pelvic pressure
- Varicose veins
- Insomnia
- Shortness of breath
- Braxton-Hicks contractions
- Full, heavy, and possibly leaky breasts
- Swelling of ankles, feet, wrists, eyelids, and face

The uterus is also putting pressure on your partner's bladder, causing a condition called "stress incontinence." This embarrassing syndrome causes mom to lose control of her bladder when she sneezes, coughs, or laughs. Though humiliating (and messy), this symptom too will disappear after baby is born. On a more serious note, the pressure on her bladder slows the flow of urine and makes the bladder lining susceptible to irritation and infection. At this late stage, something as simple as an untreated UTI can cause your partner to start preterm labor, so it is important she be on the lookout for signs of one.

Another development you are likely to notice this month is the presence of spider and varicose veins on her legs, breasts, and even her face. The appearance of these veins are a side effect of a circulatory system that has increased its blood supply between 45 and 50 percent. To accommodate the extra blood, mom's veins have expanded. But some veins have defective valves that result in visible blue varicose veins—and hemorrhoids, another type of varicose vein. Spider veins, too, are a common side effect of an increased blood supply. They are usually visible on mom's arms, chest, and face and will disappear after the birth, when mom's blood supply returns to normal.

Another side effect of mom's increased blood supply and overall fluid retention is swelling of the face, eyelids, wrists, feet, and ankles. Swelling is usually at its worst first thing in the morning when fluids have had a chance to pool in these areas. But after mom moves around, drinks water (8 to 10 glasses a day), and uses the bathroom, she should notice a decrease in swelling. Standing, sitting, or lying down for too long will increase swelling, so encourage your partner to shift position every hour or so. If her face or feet look suddenly and exceptionally puffy, she should call her doctor, as this can be a sign of preeclampsia.

In addition to feeling heavy and swollen this month, mom is also likely to have even more trouble taking deep breaths. As her uterus pushes up against her diaphragm—shifting it 1½ inches upward—tremendous pressure is put on her lungs, making it difficult to

ⓘ PREGNANCY FACT

Your baby will make movements that feel like pushes or nudges, though he may surprise you now and then with a kick or punch that you can actually see from the outside. You may even be able to feel where your baby's head and buttocks are if you press the right areas. If you are especially curious, ask your doctor to explain your baby's position, because she will be able to tell by either ultrasound or physical exam.

suck in satisfying amounts of air. It can feel scary, but both mom and baby are getting enough oxygen. Surges of progesterone have helped mom's lung capacity expand and she is, in fact, taking in more oxygen per breath than before she was pregnant.

Finally, expect your partner to gain another 4 pounds this month, for a total of 21 to 25 pounds so far. The extra weight, blood, and other fluids will cause her to tire easily after normal activities, such as grocery shopping, walking the dog, or preparing a meal. In addition, she is probably starting to be so uncomfortable that she has trouble sleeping through the night. Therefore, your partner will feel fatigued much of the time, similar to how she was feeling in the first trimester.

WHAT'S HAPPENING TO BABY

The last trimester is an incredible time of growth for baby. He is gaining about half an ounce every day—which adds up to nearly half a pound a week. By the end of the month, your baby will weigh between 4½ and 6 pounds, and be up to 18 inches long! As a result, space is at a premium in mom's belly. Your baby's kicking and jabbing will be replaced by wriggling and squirming. When timed right, dad might be able to feel and even see baby moving by watching mom's abdomen.

One movement dad definitely cannot feel is baby's increased bouts of the hiccups. As he practices breathing, your little one inhales mouthfuls of amniotic fluid. His diaphragm responds by moving up and down, resulting in hiccups. Your partner will feel these as tiny bursts of activity. All of this breathing is good practice for your baby's still-developing lungs. They are not quite ready for the outside world, and if your child was born today, he would still require breathing assistance from a ventilator and about a 6-week

---

🔍 DID YOU KNOW?

Some forms of exercise are safe bets for mom throughout pregnancy, such as walking, swimming, and prenatal yoga. However, some women find they are able to continue to jog or do aerobics if they were extremely physically active before becoming pregnant. Whatever exercise mom can still do, be sure to do something active together for at least 30 minutes each day, but stop immediately if she experiences painful contractions, bleeding, or becomes overheated and light-headed.

---

stint in the NICU. Even so, babies born at this stage in pregnancy have an excellent chance of survival with little risk of developing long-term complications.

Though it is relieving to know your baby would be OK if born this month, he still has a long way to go developmentally before he is ready to face the world. If you are having a boy, his testicles are still making their journey through his abdomen to descend into the scrotum. And if you are expecting a girl, her labia is still too small to cover her fully formed clitoris. In addition, baby has a considerable amount of brain development yet to accomplish. And unless your baby is oversized, these next several weeks are when he makes his last push to increase the fat stores that will help regulate his body temperature outside the womb.

WHAT TO EXPECT
DR.S VISITS

After this appointment, your partner's doctor will schedule

her for prenatal checkups once every two weeks. This month, she can expect the usual testing, including the urine sample, physical, and hearing the fetal heartbeat. Her doctor will also check her hands, face, feet, and ankles for swelling, and inspect any varicose veins. He will still be concerned about preeclampsia or early labor.

In addition, two new tests are likely to occur this month:

Abdominal exam: The height of mom's uterus from her pelvic bone to the top of her uterus will be measured this month. Interestingly, this number corresponds to the number of weeks pregnant she is. For example, when mom is 33 weeks along, the distance between her pubic bone and the top of her uterus will be 33 centimeters.

Kick counts: Your partner will be asked to count the number of times she feels baby move in a day. She should be able to detect 10 movements within a 2-hour period. If she is unable to detect at least 10 distinct movements in that time, call the doctor. It could indicate that baby is in distress.

✚ HEALTH CONCERNS

It is not safe for mom to take Echinacea. This is especially true during the third trimester, because Echinacea can stimulate contractions strong enough to induce preterm labor. Also, the immune system makes adjustments to support pregnancy and Echinacea can negatively interfere with those changes. If mom gets a cold, stick to orange juice and get lots of rest.

What's Happening: Dad

Third Trimester

By the eighth month of pregnancy, dad may feel like he is running on pure adrenaline and anxiety—existing solely to keep everyone sane and to get the house ready for baby. There are few conversations that do not include the words "once the baby comes."

WHAT DAD IS THINKING AND FEELING

An old Swedish proverb states, "Worry often gives a small thing a big shadow." This is an idea every father-to-be can relate to, especially in the eighth month when it seems like your life is dictated by three recurring themes: your lack of control over the health of mom and baby during labor and delivery, your uncertain future as a parent, and your reluctance to part with your old life. These feelings are normal as childbirth and fatherhood draw near, but they make baby's arrival loom large and overshadow every action and thought you have.

Getting through this period will be a lot easier if you start trusting the people around you that are going to make the birth of your child as safe and positive an experience as possible. Now is a good time, for example, to remind yourself that you trust your partner. You trust that she has managed her pregnancy these last 8 months with care and diligence. Trust that the childbirth class you are enrolled

+ HEALTH CONCERNS

Most babies produce at least four detectable movements per hour. These can include kicks, punches, hiccups, and other movements that are discernible to your partner. If your baby is not very active in the womb, she will still be healthy at birth. However, if you feel like baby is too still, mom should have a small glass of juice or water and lie on her left side for 30 to 60 minutes. If two hours have passed and she hasn't felt at least 10 movements, give your doctor a call so that you can get an immediate checkup.

in is giving mom the skills to manage the pain of labor. Trust that her doctor—who has been her pregnancy guide for many months now—is well-trained and capable of handling any emergency that may come up during the delivery. In sum, the best way for you to deal with feeling out of control is to trust that others are capable of running the show when you cannot.

Letting go of control may feel a bit like surrender, but they are not the same thing. It might be hard to see that when you feel as though your entire life has been surrendered to pregnancy—and soon to parenthood. But learning to trust others is important to keeping your sanity intact. Remind yourself that this is the first of many times in your life as a father when you will have no control and will need to lean on others for support and guidance. Take comfort in knowing that every father who came before you has had the same exact doubts. They learned quickly, as you will too, that fatherhood can only be learned by doing. This month, practice trusting that once baby is born, a combination of preparation and instincts will kick in as you and your partner figure out how to be parents together.

THINGS DAD SHOULD KNOW

The third trimester has its own important set of terms that dad should know for when mom goes into labor. Most of these concepts will be discussed at one of your partner's remaining prenatal appointments. Learning them now will help you engage in meaningful dialogue with the doctor about any concerns you have over the next several weeks.

Anterior: Baby is presenting face down for delivery

APGAR: Stands for Appearance, Pulse, Grimace, Activity, and Respiration. Baby is given a score between 1 and 10 in the first few minutes after birth to evaluate his overall health

Back labor: Labor pain that is concentrated in mom's lower back

Bloody show: Seepage of blood and mucus from the vagina—may indicate mom is losing her mucus plug

Breech presentation: when baby's rear end or feet are facing downwards

Cephalopelvic Disproportion (CPD): When mom's pelvis is too small for baby to fit through

Cervidil: A medication given to ready the cervix before mom is induced into labor

Cesarean section: Surgical delivery of a baby

DID YOU KNOW?

Some time before mom goes into labor she may pass what is called "bloody show." It can appear in the toilet or in her underwear. This happens when the mucus plug that blocks the cervical opening falls out as a result of her body preparing for labor. Her cervix will start to thin out, which will loosen the plug enough for it to become dislodged. This does not necessarily mean that she is going into labor—bloody show can happen up to 2 weeks before labor starts. When this occurs, she should let your doctor know, however.

Complete breech: Baby is presenting rear-end down with legs crossed, making vaginal delivery impossible

Crowning: When baby's head is visible outside of mom's vagina

Dilation: The number of centimeters mom's cervix has opened in preparation for baby's birth. The cervix must be 10 centimeters dilated before baby can pass through

Effacement: The thinning of the cervix in preparation for birth. When mom begins to push, she will be 100 percent effaced.

Engaged: When baby has dropped head first into mom's pelvis and is ready for delivery.

Epidural: Pain medication inserted through a catheter near mom's spinal cord

Episiotomy: A surgical cut at the back of the vagina to prevent mom from tearing during delivery

Failure to progress: When labor stops moving forward toward delivery

Forceps: Large tongs used by the doctor to help guide baby's head out of the birth canal

Frank breech: Baby is presenting rear-end-down with his legs running up the front of his body and his feet above his head

Induction of labor: Labor that is brought on by medications that encourage effacement and stimulate contractions.

Lightening: When baby drops into mom's pelvis and is engaged for delivery

Mucus plug: Collection of bodily secretions that build up over the course of pregnancy to "plug" up the cervix. Some time before labor begins mom will lose her mucus plug. It looks like a gooey ball of mucus and light pink blood. Its loss does not necessarily signify that labor has begun.

Oxytocin: Hormone that stimulates contractions and breast milk production

Perineum: Part of the body between the vagina and rectum that stretches during delivery or is cut during an episiotomy

Posterior: Baby is presenting face down for delivery

Postpartum: After baby is born

At this point in pregnancy, 75 percent of women will experience moderate to severe bouts of insomnia. This is due to frequent trips to the bathroom during the night, inability to get comfortable, vivid dreams, and anxiety. When mom is dealing with insomnia, it is important to address the causes instead of trying to force the result (sleep). Some tips include not eating too close to bed time, running mom a warm bath, and limiting her fluid intake a couple of hours before she gets into bed.

Post-term: Pregnancy that continues 2 weeks or more past the due date

Preterm: Babies born before 37 weeks

Transverse: Baby is positioned horizontally inside the uterus

Vacuum extractor: Labor tool that attaches to baby's head to help guide him out of the birth canal

Vaginal Birth After Cesarean (VBAC): When a woman who has had a previous Cesarean delivery gives birth vaginally

HELPFUL HINTS FOR DAD

Figuring out how to have safe, satisfying, and regular sex with a pregnant partner is a big challenge for dad at this point. It is likely that even if your partner is not in the mood for much of her pregnancy, you have not given up hope for a decent sex life. You can count yourself among the legions of expectant fathers who are at a loss for how to have a sex life with a pregnant partner. The following techniques may help get you closer more often.

Women need a lot more to get turned on than men, and this is especially true when they are pregnant. To warm your partner up, start with a sensual massage. Pour a little massage oil in your hands and rub together to heat. (Just be sure to avoid using certain oils that can stimulate contractions, such as jasmine or fennel.) Then, massage your partner from top to bottom while she is laying on her side. Wash your hands and switch to water-based lubricant, and surprise her with a vaginal massage.

Communicating your desires to your partner in a gentle, soft way can also get her in the mood. Tell her what you would like to do to various parts of her body while expressing your attraction to her new, voluptuous figure. Remind her of your favorite shared sexual experiences, and let her know you are willing to try different positions until you find one that is comfortable for her. Suggest that she try being on top. This angle allows her to control the depth of penetration and keeps her off her back, which is uncomfortable at this point. You can also suggest that she get on her hands and knees, while you penetrate her from behind. This is another ideal position when back pain is an issue. Again, your partner can control the depth of penetration by pulling away or leaning back. This position may get tiring, though, depending on the size of your partner's belly. Another way to try it is with your partner lying on her side while you shallowly enter her from behind. This is also a good position for when back pain, belly size, and joint point rule out other positions. Finally, you can experiment with your partner lying on her side at the edge of the bed, with you standing behind her. Wedge a pillow beneath your partner's side so that she is not lying on her back. Help her scoot her bottom to the edge of the bed and let her knees rest over your shoulders. This allows for maximum penetration, so go easy. Let your partner guide you and be willing to go slow and switch positions if she becomes uncomfortable. Hopefully, your partner's appreciation for your ingenuity will pay off with more regular bouts of sexual intimacy.

COMMON QUESTIONS THAT DADS HAVE

As the birth day gets closer, your list of questions is likely getting longer. Here are some that might be on your mind this month.

Are there certain risk factors for developing preeclampsia? Yes. While doctors are unsure why only some women develop it, there are certain criteria that increase the risk. If your partner is obese, has chronic high blood pressure, diabetes, kidney disease, an autoimmune disease, if she is carrying more than one fetus, if she is younger than 20 or older than 40, if this is her first pregnancy, or if she or a relative has had preeclampsia all influence whether she will develop the condition.

Can my partner take ibuprofen for back pain? No. Ibuprofen is not recommended during pregnancy, especially this late in one. When taken after 32 weeks, non-steroidal anti-inflammatory drugs (NSAIDs) can damage baby's arteries and kidneys. Therefore, it is best that mom manage pain by sticking to acetaminophen, massage, hot and cold compresses, and lots of rest.

Since my partner is pregnant during flu season, is it OK if she takes Echinacea? No. Echinacea is not recommended during pregnancy because it can stimulate contractions that lead to premature labor. In addition, mom's immune system is already suppressed so her body does not reject the fetus—Echinacea may interfere with that process.

ⓘ **PREGNANCY FACT**

An important development has occurred—your baby's immune system has matured and is able to fight off mild infections on its own. This was made possible by antibodies passed on from your partner as well as increased white blood cell production by your baby's bone marrow, spleen, and thymus. He will be born with a natural immunity to some viruses and will acquire others from mom if she breast-feeds him. Breast milk contains powerful antibodies, other proteins, and immune cells that help strengthen your baby.

Is it safe for my partner to donate blood? No. Your partner should not donate blood while pregnant. Though her body is producing up to 50 percent more blood than before she was pregnant, mom and baby need every drop. If mom donated blood she would deprive baby of much-needed oxygen. Besides, blood banks will not allow pregnant women to donate blood anyway.

I don't want my wife eating food heated in a microwave, because I am concerned it will harm our baby. Is this true? There is no evidence to support that food cooked in a microwave is harmful to a developing fetus. However, if you do heat food in a microwave, make sure to keep it out of plastic containers as these have been shown to leak dangerous substances called endocrine disrupters.

Is it OK to perform oral sex on my partner at this point in her pregnancy? Yes, oral sex is safe throughout pregnancy. However, take care not to blow into your partner's vagina. Though rare, it can cause an embolism (air bubble) to develop

+ HEALTH CONCERNS

An episiotomy is a small incision made in mom's perineum during delivery. It is usually done in emergency situations when baby's head is too large to fit through the vagina. The majority of women will tear during vaginal delivery—the tear can range from tiny to relatively large. Both natural tears and episiotomies make for a painful recovery, but the choice is yours and mom's (barring an emergency), so be sure to educate yourself, let your doctor know your preference, and include it in your birth plan.

that can be fatal to the baby.

Is it safe for my partner to swallow semen? Yes, as long as you do not have any sexually transmitted diseases. However, your partner may have a resurgence in nausea this month and may not want to swallow—so don't take it personally.

Since my partner has trouble getting comfortable during intercourse, is it OK to use sex toys? Vibrators and dildos are generally safe during pregnancy, but must be clean and should never be inserted too deeply. In some rare cases, vibrators have been known to injure a pregnant woman's cervix, rupture the amniotic sac, or stimulate contractions, leading to preterm labor. Therefore, if you do add sex toys, reserve them for shallow or external use only.

HOW DAD CAN DEAL

Whether or not you are the "touchy-feely" type, you will probably need support this month. As baby's birth gets closer, you are likely to doubt your ability to be a good and competent father. Ignoring these insecurities is unlikely to silence them. It can help to talk to a male friend about them. Sometimes, just hearing yourself state concerns out loud is enough to realize how off-base they are. Though some men are not comfortable talking about their feelings, studies repeatedly show that men who do are more confident in their ability to handle fatherhood.

Moreover, men who discuss their hopes and fears are more likely to have realistic expectations for fatherhood. This is important to note, because much of third trimester anxiety occurs as a result of having impossible expectations. For example, dad may expect to immediately bond with baby—but in reality, it takes days, weeks, or even months before you forge a genuine connection to your child.

Though there may not be an immediate solution to some problems—such as getting enough time off from work or finding

DID YOU KNOW?

Lightening is when baby drops into the pelvic cavity in preparation for birth. This can happen 4 weeks before labor or just a few hours before labor begins. If it happens sooner, mom will have an easier time breathing, heartburn is lessened, appetite returns, and mom's organs are less crowded. However, once baby drops, mom will need to urinate as often as every 45 minutes. She may also experience rectal discomfort from the pressure. No matter how she feels, lightening is an exciting sign that your baby is almost ready to come.

+ HEALTH CONCERNS

There are some cases in which a woman should not breast-feed; for example, if she takes medications like sedatives, antidepressants, or lithium (check with your doctor about others). If she is HIV positive, or if she is using drugs or alcohol, she can pass harmful substances to the baby. If any of these apply to your partner, she is doing the right thing by abstaining from breast-feeding. She will still be able to forge an intimate bond with your baby when feeding him formula from a bottle.

affordable childcare—talking them through will help you shoulder these burdens and might reveal tips or tricks that have helped others cope.

HOW DAD CAN HELP

Since more than 40 percent of Americans rely on herbal remedies to treat illness, it is possible your partner uses teas or supplements to deal with ailments such as gas, nausea, or congestion. However, at this late stage in her pregnancy she should avoid certain herbs and teas because they can harm baby or cause mom to go into early labor.

Help mom stay safe by reminding her to skip teas and supplements with the following ingredients:

- Blue and black cohosh
- Ephedra
- Willow bark
- Dong quai
- Rosemary oil

- Sassafras
- Buckthorn
- Senna
- Sage
- Tansy
- Coltsfoot
- Mugwort
- Comfrey
- Psillium seed
- Feverfew
- Yarrow
- Ginko
- St. John's Wort
- Echinacea
- Safflower
- Pennyroyal leaf
- Cascara sagrada
- Slippery elm

HOW DAD CAN BE INVOLVED

Helping mom create a birth plan is a great way for dad to stay in the loop this month. This simple document is an outline describing mom's preferences for labor and delivery. Items to include in the plan are who will be in attendance, preferred labor tools, if and when to administer pain medication, and what mom expects to happen after giving birth.

The birth plan should be customized and well-thought out, but flexibility is often the most important component. Sometimes, aspects of the birth plan become unrealistic during a medical emergency. Plus, you must allow for the possibility that mom might change her mind when labor actually begins—especially regarding pain relief!

A birth plan should take into account the following preferences:

Where do we want our baby to be born? Birth is no longer just for hospitals. Birthing centers and home births are increasingly popular, though reserved for only the most routine deliveries. You and your partner should consider whether you are prepared for a home birth, if you have established a relationship with a particular birthing center, and how you feel about delivering your baby in the hospital. If mom's pregnancy has been at all abnormal, it is best to deliver in a hospital.

Where will mom do early labor? Many women prefer to stay out of the hospital for as long as possible. They may want to manage early labor at home where they are more comfortable. Early labor can be managed at home by taking walks, warm baths, and having access to her favorite food and drink.

When does my partner want to go to the hospital or birthing center? Your partner may want to do the majority of her labor at home if this is not her first pregnancy. However, if this is her first baby she may want to get to the hospital as soon as they will take her.

What tools does mom want handy during labor? Examples of labor tools include a tennis ball, a sock stuffed with uncooked rice, a yoga ball, CD player, favorite CDs, portable DVD player with movies or TV shows, essential oils, candles, photos of older children or pets, and other personal items that will help mom relax.

Who does mom want with her during labor? Your partner may want one or all of the following people nearby as she labors: best friend, sister, mother, doula, midwife, or older children.

What are mom's labor preferences if she is in the hospital? Get your partner thinking about whether she will want to be walking around or if she thinks she will able to eat or drink. She'll also need to decide if she will allow fetal monitoring devices, if she will want labor to progress naturally even it takes a long time, and if she is OK with being induced. Usually, when the doctor suggests

> ### ⓘ PREGNANCY FACT
>
> If either parent has a congenital heart defect, your OB-GYN may recommend a specialist who can perform a fetal echocardiogram. This is performed the same way as the ultrasound, but zooms in on your baby's heart. It is read by a pediatric cardiologist. Fetal echocardiograms are good for detecting glaring problems in utero, which can help everyone be prepared when baby is born. If a defect is detected, your doctor will request that a pediatric cardiologist be present at the birth to assess your baby immediately.

induction it is for a medical emergency. It is often to allow mom to have a vaginal delivery instead of a Cesarean section. Induction medications can cause contractions that are more intense than those that occur naturally, and inductions that do not progress in a timely manner often end in Cesarean deliveries.

What are mom's preferences during delivery? Does she want to be allowed to push for as long as is safe for baby? Does she want to push while squatting, lying down, or sitting on the edge of a chair? Will she want to have a mirror present to watch delivery? Will she want to touch baby's head when it crowns? Will she want you to "catch" the baby when he comes out? Will she want to see the placenta after it is pushed out or hold the baby immediately after giving birth? Her answers to each of these questions will inform her birth plan.

Can mom refuse an episiotomy? In some cases, a small incision is necessary to allow enough room for baby's head to fit through the vagina. If mom is adamantly opposed to having an

✖ TIPS & ADVICE

> Mom's traveling days are over, due to the danger that she may go into labor at any time. She should avoid long car, bus, and train rides, as sitting for long periods of time will not only be uncomfortable but will increase swelling. If she travels for work, she should pass that baton to someone else. If you've got the itch to get away before baby comes, make the most of a local weekend getaway.

episiotomy she should include it in her birth plan. If she refuses one, however, she should be prepared for her perineum to tear during a vaginal delivery.

Does mom want pain medication during labor? This is usually the part of the birth plan women have the strongest opinions about. Remind your partner not to get too attached to any preference. Many women who say "No" to pain medication on their birth plans change their minds once true labor begins. On the other hand, many women who say "Yes" later realize they can do labor without it and decide to forgo the epidural. Types of medications preferred should also go in the birth plan.

What other preferences should go in the birth plan? Think about whether dad will want to cut the umbilical cord. Also to be considered is whether mom wants to try nursing immediately, or if the medical staff should clean baby up first. Does mom want baby to get formula while in the hospital? Will you want pictures or video of the birth? Will you want to store your baby's cord blood? Will you want your son circumcised? The answers to each of these questions should be in your birth plan.

DAD'S RESPONSIBILITIES

This month, your job is to have hospital bags packed and ready to go in the event that baby comes early. Items to include are a few days' supply of clothes, pajamas, labor tools mom wants on-hand, an outfit for baby to wear home, and important documents (such as insurance cards, birth plan, and ID cards). Keep the bags near the front door so you don't have to frantically search for them.

"Everything about woman is a riddle."
~ Friedrich Nietzsche

Notes . . . .

Lunar Month

Nine

Third Trimester

Lunar Month nine . . . . 🦆

MONTHLY TO-DO LISTS

- ❏ Help stock the nursery with diapers, wipes, and other necessities
- ❏ Help mom rein in her nesting instinct
- ❏ Assemble the crib
- ❏ Install the car seat
- ❏ Finish childbirth preparation classes
- ❏ Pre-register at the hospital
- ❏ Remind your employer that mom is due this month
- ❏ Start a college fund for baby
- ❏ Help your partner avoid long-distance travel
- ❏ Remind your partner to get up slowly to prevent passing out
- ❏ Help your partner eat foods low in sodium to avoid unnecessary swelling
- ❏ Be on the lookout for baby's movements through mom's stomach
- ❏ Stay calm, and be ready to go!

MY PERSONAL CHECKLIST:

- ❏ ....
- ❏ ....
- ❏ ....

MY HOPES FOR THIS MONTH:

....

....

....

....

....

....

....

What's Happening: Mom & Baby

Lunar Month 9

Third Trimester

WHAT'S HAPPENING TO MOM

MOM'S Symptoms

- **Vaginal discharge that contains mucus and blood**
- **Constipation**
- **Heartburn and gas**
- **Nausea and congestion**
- **Back pain and/or sciatica**
- **Headaches and dizziness**
- **Shortness of breath**

The ninth month tends to drag on for mom, because she has reached the height of discomfort. Her uterus is putting pressure on nearly every organ and bone in its vicinity. Swelling has increased, squeezing nerves in her back, buttocks, ankles, wrists, and hands. The good news is that many of these symptoms will be relieved toward the end of the month when baby drops—called lightening. But in the meantime, the weight of mom's uterus and its contents—all 11 to 13 pounds of baby, placenta, and amniotic fluid—makes your partner feel cranky, tired, and ready for pregnancy to be over.

Now tucked up under her rib cage, the pressure of her uterus forces her ribs out and her diaphragm

MOM'S
Symptoms

- Leg cramps
- Carpal tunnel syndrome
- Swelling of extremities
- Varicose veins, hemorrhoids
- Insomnia and fatigue
- Braxton-Hicks contractions
- Frequent urination
- Leaky, full breasts
- Clumsiness
- Increased or decreased appetite
- Sensation that baby is squirming and wriggling
- Onset of "nesting" instinct

up. This continues to make it difficult for mom to take deep breaths as her diaphragm crowds the space where her lungs normally sit. Shallow breathing coupled with extra blood diverted to the fetus may cause your partner to feel dizzy or light-headed. She might even feel as though oxygen is not reaching her brain—but it is. However, pooling fluid puts her at risk for passing out if she stands up too quickly, so remind her to take her time doing so.

Besides causing mom to feel dizzy, pooling fluids can bring about edema, a condition in which the ankles, feet, hands, wrists, and face swell. Though normal, edema triggers other painful conditions by putting pressure on nerves. One is carpal tunnel syndrome (CTS). As fluid builds up in the carpal tunnel inside mom's wrists, it puts pressure on the median nerve and causes her hands to ache, tingle, or go completely numb. Since swelling is usually worse first thing in the morning and at night, moms who develop CTS are encouraged to wear a soft wrist brace on the affected side while sleeping. If the condition persists throughout the day, mom should stop using her hands for repetitive motion activities, such as typing, doing dishes, or sweeping. She should also avoid foods high in sodium, drink 8 to 10 glasses of water a day, and elevate hands and feet

ⓘ PREGNANCY FACT

Congratulations! You are in the final leg of pregnancy. You have been through a lot, dad: body changes, emotional upheaval, mood swings, and the mounting expectation of who this tiny person will turn out to be. Try to savor these last few weeks together without baby. Spend time being intimate with mom, because she will be back to her old self in just a few months.

whenever possible. Edema worsens after sitting in one position for too long, so long-distance travel is not recommended.

Another reason to stick close to home is that the hormone relaxin is flooding your partner's body, causing her joints to loosen up. This makes her feel achy and sore all over. As a result, mom's hips, lower back, and pelvis hurt—they may even feel as though they are separating from her body. This sensation is not only uncomfortable, but leads to clumsiness. Therefore, she needs to be extra-careful when taking the stairs or getting in and out of the car as she will become prone to falling.

WHAT'S HAPPENING TO BABY

This is a big month for your baby. By the end of it, baby is considered full-term. As a result, most of her physical development will be completed within the next few weeks, with the exception of her brain and digestive tract, which continue to develop after birth. Baby's main job until she is born to is to add fat and finish developing her lungs. Indeed, her greatest gains are made over the next 3 to 4 weeks, when she will add about a half a pound a week to her little frame. By the end of the month, she will weigh between 6½ and 7½

> ### 🔍 DID YOU KNOW?
>
> Each time you see your doctor, he will check for baby's presentation, or birth position. By now, she is probably head-down, the ideal position for vaginal delivery. If this is your first baby, she will likely stay in the position she is in now. Women who have had other children sometimes find that baby may change position up to the last week of pregnancy. If your doctor has difficulty determining your baby's presentation by external exam, she may do a vaginal exam to feel which part of baby is closest to the exit.

pounds and may be up to 20 inches long.

Baby's increase in size makes his living quarters cramped and difficult to move around in. Therefore, mom will experience his movements as squirming, wriggling, and rolling, since he no longer has enough space to kick or punch. These kinds of movements are pronounced and sometimes very forceful. You might even be able to see baby pushing out through mom's abdomen during highly active periods.

Even when baby is resting, though, his body is preparing for birth. Over the next 3 to 4 weeks, his body sheds most of the lanugo, the fine hair that covers his body and the wax-like vernix caseosa that will help him ease through the birth canal. In addition, he can open and close his eyes—at this point he can even see light that filters in through mom's uterus, and may turn away from it. He also continues to practice swallowing and breathing, and his kidneys and liver are functioning well enough to process and rid his body of waste.

As he swallows his own sterile urine, lanugo, discarded skin cells, and amniotic fluid, his first stool—called meconium—is forming in his intestines. Despite all of this, his digestive tract will not be fully mature until he is 3 or 4 years old.

Finally, your baby's lungs continue to produce surfactant—a substance that prevents his lungs from sticking together when breathing. This is the most important reason why you want your baby to remain in utero until he reaches full term. Sufficient production of surfactant is required for his lungs to inflate. Indeed, most babies who are born preterm end up in the NICU due to insufficient lung-development. However, babies born any time this month have an excellent chance of surviving and thriving.

WHAT TO EXPECT
DR.S VISITS

Your partner will see her doctor twice this month. During each appointment, she will provide a urine sample, have her weight and blood pressure checked, and hear baby's heartbeat.

The doctor will also ask about the frequency of baby's movements. Some other tests to expect include:

Abdominal exam: The height of mom's uterus from her pelvic bone to the top of her uterus will be measured. The doctor will also check baby's position by pressing down on mom's abdomen. If she cannot tell from an external exam, she may do a vaginal exam as well.

Ultrasound or sonogram: An ultrasound will be performed only if mom has health problems or if the doctor is concerned with baby's position, development, or with the amount of amniotic fluid.

Group B strep test: A swab will be taken to your partner's rec-

+ HEALTH CONCERNS

Your doctor will monitor the level of amniotic fluid surrounding the baby. If the fluid level is too low, mom could be in for an early or complicated delivery. The main concern is that the lack of protective solution will cause the umbilical cord to become compressed. Thus, your doctor may decide to induce labor or perform a C-section.

tum and vagina to test for the Group B streptococci (GBS) bacteria. Though harmless to mom, GBS can have devastating consequences if contracted by baby during delivery. If mom is like 1 in 4 pregnant women who carry the bacteria, she will be treated with antibiotics during delivery to prevent transmission to baby.

Nonstress test: This non-invasive test requires mom to sit in a chair or lie on her side while hooked up to a machine that monitors baby's heartbeat as well as uterine contractions. She will have a snack before the test to help wake baby up. This test is done when mom has health problems such as gestational diabetes or hypertension or if there has been a drop off in baby's movements.

Biophysical profile (BPP): BPP is a combination ultrasound and nonstress test. It gauges whether baby is receiving enough oxygen and determines whether baby should be delivered early.

Contraction stress test: This test is conducted on women with high-risk pregnancies to determine whether baby can handle the stress of labor. Mom will be hooked up to a device that measures uterine contractions and baby's heartbeat. If she is not having contractions, mom may be injected with synthetic oxytocin—which promotes contractions—and monitored for up to 2 hours.

What's Happening: Dad

Third Trimester

This month is all about gearing up to meet your baby. Getting ready includes staying positive, finishing any projects leftover from last month, attending the last few childbirth education classes, and keeping mom relaxed as you both wait for labor to begin.

WHAT DAD IS THINKING AND FEELING

These days you are probably all over the map. One day you are excited to meet your child—the next you are panic-stricken and rethinking this whole "have a kid" thing. Hopefully, the nerves and guilt do not outweigh the number of times you notice an extra spring in your step or a flutter in your chest when thoughts turn to the day your partner will give birth to your baby.

The ninth month is a charged time for dads. Even if your partner's due date is weeks away, each day feels as though it could be the day. As only 5 percent of babies are born on their actual due date, there is a good chance you could meet your child sooner than you thought. Ninety-five percent of babies are born either before or after their estimated due date (EDD), though most first-time moms give birth up to two weeks after their EDD. Because of the unpredictability of birth, it is smart to be prepared for your partner to go into labor at any time.

✖ FOOD FOR THOUGHT

In addition to feeding baby after he is born, you and your partner will have to deal with feeding yourselves. Therefore, start collecting menus from your favorite restaurants that deliver. Put them in a folder in a drawer in the kitchen. Sometimes it is just easier to have a pizza delivered than anything else. Also, ask friends and family to come over for a cooking party where each person prepares a dish for you to freeze and have ready to prepare after your baby comes home.

Being prepared is not just having suitcases packed and ready to go—it is also about getting into a mindset that facilitates a calm, confident zone in which mom can seek comfort in these last weeks of pregnancy. Learning to be Zen about labor and delivery is not an easy task for either parent, but it is especially difficult for mom this month. Therefore, work to make the home environment as peaceful as possible by keeping your fears from her.

A common feeling for men to experience this month is guilt. As labor and delivery loom closer, dad starts to feel guilty for putting his partner through such a painful and dramatic experience. You may even be consumed by regret for impregnating your partner in the first place. No matter how awful your partner feels, though, it is not likely that she would want to trade places. Even in the midst of the most uncomfortable pregnancy, labor, and delivery conditions, your partner feels lucky that she will give birth. Chalk this up to the fact that women are predisposed to the task of childbirth—just part of the mystery and wonder of the process.

THINGS DAD SHOULD KNOW

Throughout this month and next, your partner will become highly motivated by the "nesting" instinct. Though she has already engaged in some of following behaviors, her personality takes a decidedly loopy turn this month. You will notice she rarely wants to leave the house, and has probably started a few massive reorganizing and cleaning projects. It is not unusual for dad to get roped into this frenetic effort to create the perfect "nest," so be ready to be assaulted with to-do lists the minute you get home from work.

Things that need to be done include:

Preparing baby's room: If the nursery is not yet ready for baby—and even if it is—mom may want to repeatedly clean the room, repaint the walls, move furniture, get new curtains, wash, dry, and fold every piece of baby's clothing, and install or remove carpet. You should take on larger projects, such as painting and assembling furniture, and let mom handle smaller projects, such as dusting and organizing.

Cleaning: For mom, the house can never be clean enough for baby. She may want to vacuum and clean the floors, cupboards, windows, and bathrooms, every other day until baby's arrival. There is no harm in this, other than exposure to harsh chemicals. Invest in non-toxic, eco-friendly cleaning products and let her go to town.

Organizing: You may come home to find that your partner has dumped the contents of your closet onto the floor. Don't worry—she is just organizing! It is common for women to unpack closets and drawers to take inventory of what treasures have collected over the years. It keeps them busy during an anxious time and satisfies their need to ready the house for baby. Though you should not interrupt

If your doctor is concerned with the health of your baby and needs information beyond that which the non-stress test can provide, she may ask mom to come in for fetal acoustical stimulation (FAS). FAS is done by placing a device on your partner's abdomen that produces vibrations that your baby should respond to. This test is valuable for determining if your baby is moving as much as he should be, and it will also give a more accurate read on baby's cardiac response to stimulation.

this process, encourage mom to stick with one room and finish what she started before moving on to the next. Otherwise, she may throw the entire house into disarray and be too overwhelmed to put it back in order.

Alphabetizing: Another common manifestation of the nesting instinct is to feel compelled to alphabetize every book, piece of mail, CD, DVD, and magazine in your house. Alphabetizing items and putting photos in chronological order is a soothing way for mom to stay busy while waiting for labor to begin. However, as with her drawer-and-closet reorganization, try to reel in how many of these projects she starts to prevent them from becoming an additional stressor.

It can be hard for dad to keep up with mom's various "emergency" projects this month. Plus, it is really frustrating to come home to a dismantled house. Try and treat it with humor, and know it will soon pass.

HELPFUL HINTS FOR DAD

You may feel overcome with your own version of the nesting instinct this month. In men this is often expressed as the urge to do something productive with your time. Keeping your hands busy discourages you from coping with stress by overeating or drinking, or even going back to smoking if you had quit during the pregnancy. It also helps prevent you from obsessing over worst-case labor and delivery scenarios.

Suggested tasks to accomplish this month include:

Install the car seat: Installing the car seat before mom goes into labor is both practical and smart. Putting it in now gives you time to practice using it so that you will be ready to drive home with baby. When installing a car seat, remember that they always go in the backseat. Infant car seats should be rear-facing until your child turns 1 and weighs 20 pounds. The seat should be secured tightly enough so it can't be moved more than an inch in any direction. If your car has side airbags in the backseat, place the car seat in the center of the seat bench. Finally, make sure the car seat sits at the proper angle so that baby's head does not roll forward, backward, or to one side. Most car seats come with an indicator that tells you when it is level. And of course, secure seatbelts, cords, or other loose items that could fall on your child.

Make arrangements for someone to care for other kids or pets during the birth: Make a plan for who will care for older children and pets when your partner goes into labor. It will be less stressful for all involved if the caretaker is someone well-known and used to household routines. It is also best if this person stays at your house until you and mom return home with your newborn.

Let your employer know you may have to go at any time: Though you told your boss about the pregnancy months ago, it is unlikely he has given it much thought since then. Now is the time to remind him that your partner is in her ninth month and that you could be called any time to get home or to the hospital.

Pre-register at the hospital: Pre-registering at the hospital saves time once mom goes into labor. This simple process takes just a few minutes and a small amount of paperwork. Your partner's doctor can provide you with the necessary form—often with a postage-paid envelope—so all you have to do is fill it out and mail it. By pre-registering, you make sure the hospital has your insurance information, knows who your partner's doctor is, is aware of any pertinent medical information, knows who your baby's pediatrician is (if you have already selected one), and when to expect mom for labor and delivery based on her EDD.

Finish up childbirth preparation classes: You should complete childbirth preparation classes this month. Attend each one, as they get progressively more informative toward the end. Most classes end with a tour of the maternity floor where your partner will deliver baby. This is usually a favorite for parents who like being able to visualize where labor and delivery will take place. The tour tends to de-escalate the anxieties they have about having their baby in a hospital.

COMMON QUESTIONS THAT DADS HAVE

What if my partner cannot get ahold of me when labor starts? Avoid this by having several ways of staying in touch. If you don't already have a cell phone, get one. Enable its Web-access features so you can check email and traffic routes. Let colleagues know you will be keeping your phone on vibrate during meetings.

When packing your labor bag for the hospital, include the following: at least two copies of your birth plan; a stopwatch to time contractions; a camera and/or video camera; important phone numbers; a stress or tennis ball for squeezing; candies to keep mom from getting thirsty; warm socks; slippers; a robe; toothbrush; hairbrush; something to hold mom's hair back; photos of other children or pets; a CD player with soothing music; a yoga ball for mom to sit on; and a mini DVD player and movies.

Above all, don't travel more than an hour from home during these last few weeks.

What if I am too squeamish to cut the umbilical cord?

Many dads think they can't handle cutting the umbilical cord, but then end up feeling emboldened by mom's bravery during childbirth and decide to do it. Others think "no problem, I can do it," only to discover they can't look at anything below mom's shoulders. You'll know in the moment what you are capable of—and your partner will be so relieved from giving birth, she will be fine with whatever you decide.

What are the chances that our baby will be stillborn?

Stillbirth occurs when a fetus dies after the 20th week of pregnancy. If your partner has gone in for her regular prenatal checkups, chances are slim that your child will be stillborn since baby's activity has been regularly monitored. Even so, there is always a tiny chance something could go horribly wrong. Researchers are stumped by what causes the majority of stillbirths, but have been able to narrow it down into 3 categories. One is birth defects,

ⓘ PREGNANCY FACT

Before your baby is born, his lungs are flat and his body must work extra hard to get blood to circulate through them. Once he is born, though, and the umbilical cord is cut, his body craves oxygen, which causes his lungs to inflate (thanks to the vital fluid called surfactant). Baby takes his first breath out of reflex and necessity. Once his lungs are inflated, the flow in the left side of your baby's heart strengthens and his circulation increases. His lungs will continue to develop throughout his infancy.

which 25 percent of stillborn babies have. Another is a defective placenta or umbilical cord which prevented them from receiving enough oxygen and/or nutrients. Finally, in some cases, mom's poor health—such as diabetes or hypertension—or drug use can lead to a stillbirth.

What is Sudden Infant Death Syndrome, and how worried should I be about it? Sudden Infant Death Syndrome (SIDS) is the unexplained death of a sleeping baby within the first year of its life. SIDS claims 2,000 infants each year. The reason is usually never determined. Thus, there is little you can do but be aware of the risks for SIDS (covered later in this book), keep secondhand smoke away from your baby, and be vigilant about your baby sleeping on his back. Just know that it is rare and push it from your mind. Instead focus on helping your partner through labor and delivery.

Will my wife really be able to lose all the weight she gained? Yes. Your partner will most likely get back to her pre-pregnancy weight within the first year after baby is born—

especially if she plans to breast-feed. Nursing a baby burns about 500 extra calories a day. This is on top of the calories she burns doing normal activities and exercising. But don't push her to lose weight. It will take her a month or more to recover from giving birth and up to a year for her hormones to return to normal.

HOW DAD CAN DEAL

Dealing with the last several weeks of pregnancy is stressful and busy, but not as much as when your newborn is actually home. In just a few weeks, you will be transformed into a family, so it's a good idea to overload on relaxation during these last few weeks of calm. Take advantage of intimate moments while it is still just you and your partner.

✚ HEALTH CONCERNS

If baby's body is putting too much pressure on the umbilical cord, it can decrease blood flow and the amount of oxygen that gets to baby. If this occurs during labor, your doctor may have mom contorting into many different positions to try to get the baby to move off the cord. Since this usually happens close to when baby is about to be born, your doctor may decide that use of forceps or a vacuum extractor is necessary. He might also skip these and do a Cesarean if your baby is still too high for them to move.

Take the pressure off the looming deadline of birth by snuggling up and watching one of these classic parenthood films:

- *Betsy's Wedding*
- *Bringing Up Baby*
- *For Keeps*
- *From Conception to Birth*
- *Knocked Up*
- *Look Who's Talking 1-4*
- *Mr. Mom*
- *Paper Moon*
- *Parenthood*
- *Raising Arizona*
- *She's Having A Baby*
- *The Champ*
- *The Parent Trap*
- *Three Men and A Baby*

HOW DAD CAN HELP

This month, you can help by spearheading the effort to find a pediatrician. This is one task you do not want to wait to tend to, because whomever you choose will be the doctor who sees your child in the hospital. If you don't pre-select a pediatrician, the hospital will send whoever is on duty when your partner gives birth. Plus, your medical insurance plan will likely have rules about coverage that will require your consideration, such as when you have to enroll your newborn and which medical groups are covered. Leaving this decision until after your son or daughter is born is likely to be expensive and stressful.

Use the following guide to help you find the right doctor for your family and insurance plan.

Talk to friends with kids: The best advertisement is a satisfied customer—so talk to friends and family with kids about their pediatrician. Ask what they like about the doctor, what her office hours are, how long she has been in practice, and how their children respond to her.

🔍 DID YOU KNOW?

At the end of Week 35, your baby will be considered full-term. This is very exciting, because it means that all of his bodily systems will be operational and able to function outside of your partner's uterus. If mom's pregnancy has been without complications and your baby is born near the end of this week, he will have an excellent of survival. He will also have an excellent chance of boarding in-room with you and mom, without requiring special medical attention.

Check with your insurance plan: There is no point in getting attached to a doctor that your insurance plan will not cover. Call your insurance provider or check their website to see if the doctors on your list are covered.

Find out if the doctors you like are accepting new patients: Next, call the doctors on your list and find out if they are accepting new patients with your insurance plan. There is no point in pursuing them if they are not.

Do a background check: Find out where a doctor got his degree and whether he has been subject to disciplinary action. To do this, contact the Federation of State Medical Boards (www.fsmb.org) or the Public Citizen's Health Research Group (www.citizen.org/hrg).

Interview your top choices: Narrow your selections down to just a couple of doctors and make appointments to interview them. Both you and your partner should be present to ask the following: How many offices do you have? How many doctors are in the group?

✖ TIPS & ADVICE

If your baby is in the posterior position when labor begins (the back of his head pressing on mom's spine), she will probably experience back labor. Back labor is severe back pain that accompanies contractions and does not let up between them. But don't worry too much—only 15 percent of babies are posterior at the start of labor and many will turn around before it is time to push. To ease the pain of back labor, have mom get on her hands and knees and do pelvic tilts. If you massage her lower back, that can also help.

Do you keep evening and Saturday hours? Who do you call in case of an after-hours emergency? Are you accepting of alternative child-rearing practices, such as exclusively breast-feeding, raising a vegetarian child, circumcising, etc.? Are you usually on schedule? Do you approach health from a holistic perspective? Are you up-to-date on the latest medical and development trends? What are your fees for well-child visits? Immunizations? Sick visits? To what age will you treat my child?

Evaluate the condition of the office: Many terrific pediatricians are supported by rude and inattentive staff. Pay attention to the front desk and nursing staff when you are there. Notice the condition of the office. Do they separate sick kids and those there for regular checkups? Is the office clean? Is staff respectful to waiting parents?

HOW DAD CAN BE INVOLVED

There is no time like the present to start saving for your child's college fund. It seems crazy to think, but your child will be graduating from high school before you know it. With college tuition and associated costs rising every year, college is one of the most expensive purchases made in one's lifetime—yet one which is well worth it. Besides opening a regular savings account that accrues interest, there are other types of accounts available to parents who want to put money aside for college tuition.

529 college savings plan: This state-sponsored savings plan allows parents to accrue up to $305,000 in an investment account toward their child's college tuition and related expenses. This plan allows you to select an investment option offered by your state that is professionally managed. Contributions to the account may be made by anyone, not just parents. Though contributions cannot be used as deductibles on your federal tax return, the money is allowed to grow tax-deferred. In addition, the Pension Protection Act of 2006 made permanent tax-free disbursements to educational institutions. However, state tax treatment varies according to where you live and must be looked into before opening an account. The money can be used at any college or university within the United States and there is no time limit for when the money must be used. Finally, the money can only be used for education, but it may be transferred to siblings or to mom or dad to use for school if the intended recipient does not need it.

529 prepaid tuition plan: Also known as a Prepaid Education Arrangement (PEA), this state-sponsored college-savings plan allows parents to buy in-state public education at current prices. In other words, purchasing a semester at your local public university at the current tuition will be honored when your child enrolls 17 or 18 years from now. This is an excellent way to lock in tuition costs, which are almost sure to rise over time. It is also a great fit for parents who live in states with excellent public schools. In some cases, the funds may be transferred for use at private or out-of-state universities, but rules depend on the state in which the plan was purchased. The money invested in this plan must be used for education. Check with your financial advisor or accountant for individual state tax laws.

Custodial account: Established under the Uniform Gift to Minors Act (UTMA) this type of account is managed by the custodian—or parent—until the child reaches 18 or 21 years old (depending on the state). Custodial funds are usually invested in mutual funds or bonds, are not tax-deferred, and must be claimed on the child's tax return. Monies earned over $1,500 annually will be taxed at your rate until your child turns 14. At this time, the Kiddie Tax rate will be applied to the funds. In addition, gifts made to the account cannot be transferred back to the parent. One advantage to donors is that gifts up to $10,000 a year may be given without paying a gift tax. Also, money may be used by the child for any purpose once he reaches legal termination age and takes over the account. A major disadvantage to this type of account, however, is that it may significantly reduce the amount of financial aid your child is eligible for receiving from a school.

ⓘ PREGNANCY FACT

Early labor is when the cervical opening goes from 0 to 3 centimeters. Contractions during early labor usually last between 30 and 60 seconds and come between 5 and 20 minutes apart. This phase of labor usually lasts the longest and is the least painful, so you and mom may want to stay home to do early labor. Your partner will be more comfortable and have more freedom. In fact, many hospitals will send her home and tell her to come back once contractions are coming more frequently and with more intensity.

As the big day approaches, you should discuss your role when mom goes into labor. Hopefully, you both learned a lot in your childbirth class, but it can help to talk it out so that you feel more prepared. In general, you should be prepared to offer emotional support and reassure mom that she is doing great. You are her coach and should remind her how and when to employ breathing techniques. You are also responsible for timing contractions and should be familiar with how to touch mom to help her relax.

Coverdell Education Savings Account (CESA) or Education IRA: Up to $2,000 a year can be invested in a CESA account. Funds may be invested in mutual funds over a long period of time and contributions may grow tax-free. Money put in the fund is not tax-deductible, but funds are not taxed when withdrawn for educational use. If not used by the time your child is 30, the funds may be transferred to a sibling or to your child's offspring. Funds may be used for any level of educational spending from grade school to university. It is important to note that contributions cannot be made to a CESA and a 529 account in the same year. Also, your child is limited to having one CESA, meaning grandma cannot open one for your child if you have already done so.

DAD'S RESPONSIBILITIES

If you have fallen behind on your getting-ready-for-baby projects, you are rapidly running out of time to accomplish them. Set aside the upcoming weekend to make sure the crib is assembled and the car seat is installed. Make sure you partner has purchased items she might not have received at her baby shower, like a breast pump, infant clothes, and a comfortable nursing chair. Finally, if you and your partner haven't yet settled on a name, give this process extra thought while there is still time. It seems hard to believe, but many couples who don't make up their mind prior to going to the hospital end up naming their child something neither of them really love. If you don't know the baby's gender, have both a girl name and a boy name ready to list on that birth certificate!

"Making a decision to have a child—it's momentous. It is to decide forever to have your heart go walking around outside your body."
~ Elizabeth Stone

Lunar Month

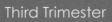

Ten

Third Trimester

MONTHLY TO-DO LISTS

- ❏ Help mom relax
- ❏ Learn to recognize pre-labor symptoms
- ❏ Start a time capsule for baby
- ❏ Make sure the house is ready and all pre-baby projects are completed
- ❏ Stick close to home
- ❏ Check in with partner several times a day when at work
- ❏ Make sure mom doesn't bathe with any essential oils
- ❏ Don't have sex with your partner after her mucus plug becomes dislodged
- ❏ Gather the phone numbers of friends and family who will need to be contacted when baby is born
- ❏ Designate someone to head up calling the list if that is how you want to spread the news

MY PERSONAL CHECKLIST:

- ❏ ....
- ❏ ....
- ❏ ....

MY HOPES FOR THIS MONTH:

....

....

....

....

....

....

....

What's Happening: Mom & Baby

Lunar Month 10

Third Trimester

WHAT'S HAPPENING TO MOM

MOM'S Symptoms

- Vaginal discharge that contains mucus and blood
- Baby dropping into pelvis
- Constipation
- Heartburn and nausea
- Gas and indigestion
- Vaginal pain
- Achy buttocks and hips
- Itchy abdomen

The 10th month of pregnancy generally lasts just two weeks until mom reaches her estimated due date. But these two weeks may feel like an eternity as she suffers multiple side effects from the 25 to 35 pounds she has gained.

Though only 6 to 8 pounds of her weight gain is fat, she feels like a whale trying to walk (or waddle). With good reason: When labor starts, your partner's uterus will weigh 20 times more than it did before she was pregnant—and this does not even include its contents! Most of the weight mom carries is focused in her abdominal area, which challenges her center of gravity and predisposes her to back pain and clumsiness.

MOM'S Symptoms

- Back pain and/or sciatica
- Headaches and dizziness
- Shortness of breath
- Leg cramps
- Carpal tunnel
- Swelling of extremities
- Varicose veins
- Hemorrhoids
- Insomnia and fatigue
- Braxton-Hicks contractions
- Frequent urination
- Leaky, full breasts
- Broken water

She is likely feeling extremely self-conscious and like she will never return to her normal size. You can help keep her self-esteem up by reminding her that very little of the weight will stick with her after the birth.

Here is how her pregnancy weight actually breaks down:

- Baby weighs 6½ to 9 pounds
- Placenta weighs 1½ to 2 pounds
- Amniotic fluid weighs 2 to 2½ pounds
- Breasts weigh 1 to 3 pounds
- Uterus weighs 2 to 2½ pounds
- Fat weighs 6 to 8 pounds
- Blood volume weighs 3 to 4 pounds
- Fluid volume weighs 2½ to 3 pounds

Although mom's weight will stabilize this month, associated aches and pains will increase. Also, her body is producing even more relaxin to ready her pelvis for expansion during delivery, which increases joint pain in her hips and abdomen. Most of these symptoms have been present for awhile but will intensify as her due date gets closer.

A new symptom this month is the development of vaginal pain. This occurs as mom's cervix begins to dilate. This pain manifests as a sharp, pinching sensation this is pretty uncomfortable. However, it is a normal part of the body's process to ready itself for delivery, and is not cause for concern.

Indeed, the body must go through many changes over the next couple weeks to prepare for childbirth. One of these changes is called lightening. This is when baby drops from being nestled under mom's rib cage into her pelvis, hopefully facing head-down. Note that it is common in first-time pregnancies for lightening to occur days or weeks before labor begins. Women who have been pregnant before may not feel baby drop until labor actually starts. Therefore, lightening is not an accurate way to gauge whether real labor has begun.

The same is true for when your partner's water breaks (fluid that results from a leaking or ruptured amniotic sac). Contrary to movies in which pregnant women ruin a pair of new shoes with a big gush of water, only 10 percent of moms experience their water breaking before labor starts. Therefore, mom should not depend on it as a sign that she is in labor. However, if your partner does notice a steady trickle of clear or yellowish fluid from her vagina—different from leukorrhea, or vaginal discharge, which will also increase this month—notify the doctor or head to the emergency room for immediate evaluation.

WHAT'S HAPPENING TO BABY

Now considered full-term, your baby is pretty much out of room in mom's uterus. He or she is truly a fully formed little person, ready to greet the world! Each day in utero is just extra time to perfect his organ functioning and a chance to put on a little more weight.

ⓘ PREGNANCY FACT

Congratulations! Your baby is now full-term. You now have no need to be concerned if mom goes into labor before the due date. You will definitely see your doctor this week for a checkup. At this appointment, you can expect an internal exam to determine if she is dilated and if effacement has begun. If your doctor detects problems with mom or baby's health, he may schedule a Cesarean section or induction. After all, at this point, all your baby's organs are fully developed, functional, and ready for life on the outside.

When he is born, your baby will weigh between 7 and 9 pounds and be 19½ to 21 inches long. He'll be attached to more than 2 feet of um-bilical cord. The placenta that has supplied him with nutrients, oxy-gen, and much-needed antibodies over the course of the pregnancy will be delivered shortly after he is, thus the term afterbirth.

WHAT TO EXPECT
DR.S VISITS

Your partner will see her doctor once a week until baby is born, and during each appointment she will provide a urine sample, have her weight and blood pressure checked, and hear baby's heartbeat. In addition, the doctor will check mom's hands, face, feet, and ankles for swelling and inspect varicose veins. The doctor will also ask about the frequency of baby's movements and inquire about mom's overall health and symptoms. It is likely that she and her doctor will go over her birth plan, so be sure to have it laid out by now.

Some additional tests to expect this month include:
Abdominal exam: Once again, the doctor will measure the height of mom's fundus. This month, her uterus will measure be-

tween 38 and 40 centimeters, corresponding with the number of weeks she has been pregnant. The doctor will also check the baby's position by feeling what his presenting part is. She does this by pressing down on mom's abdomen. If she cannot tell from an external exam, the doctor may do a vaginal exam as well.

Nonstress test: Mom may be asked to do another nonstress test. As you recall from last month, this non-invasive test is conducted in the doctor's office. Mom sits in a comfortable chair or lies on her side while hooked up to a machine that monitors baby's heartbeat and uterine contractions. Mom will be asked to have a snack before the test to help wake up the baby. This test is done when mom has health problems, such as gestational diabetes or hypertension, or if there has been a drop off in baby's movements.

Biophysical profile (BPP): BPP is a combination of the ultrasound and nonstress test. It gauges whether baby is receiving enough oxygen and determines whether the baby is thriving or should be de-

🔍 DID YOU KNOW?

If your partner's pregnancy is without complications and your doctor has not told you to avoid sex and orgasms—go for it. You will have to be creative but, at this point, the most comfortable positions tend to be spooning, mom on top, and mom on her hands and knees. You may be concerned about how having an orgasm affects the baby; during an orgasm, baby feels something similar to the Braxton-Hicks contractions he's used to by now. There is little risk for orgasm inducing labor if the pregnancy has been normal.

✖ TIPS & ADVICE

> Slow, deep breathing is an effective way for mom to become grounded and more relaxed between contractions. It also provides oxygen to the muscles so they can function more effectively, and there will be less pain. Breathe in deeply through your nose while counting to 10. Hold for a few seconds, and then exhale for a 10-count. Try to expel every bit of breath from your lungs. You should both practice deep breathing several times daily so that you are able to easily fall into a pattern once true labor starts.

livered early. It will be conducted as needed until the baby is born.

Contraction stress test: If your partner has had a high-risk pregnancy, she will undergo this test again. It evaluates how well the baby will be able to handle the stress of labor. During this test, mom will be hooked up to a device that measures uterine contractions, as well as baby's heartbeat. If mom is not having contractions, the doctor may ask her to stimulate her nipples. This causes her body to release oxytocin, a contraction-stimulating hormone. If this does not work, the doctor may inject her with synthetic oxytocin and monitor her for up to 2 hours.

Doppler sonography: This test uses the same equipment as an ultrasound, but it measures blood flow to the umbilical cord as well as to baby's organs and limbs. It can also determine the health of the placenta and help the doctor decide whether mom should be induced or have a Cesarean section prior to her due date.

What's Happening: Dad

Lunar Month 10

Third Trimester

The 10th month is a nail-biter. You have no doubt that by the end of the month, your newborn will be here! With most of the big responsibilities completed, each day is an exercise in passing time until mom goes into labor. This can be a maddening way to live, fraught with nervous excitement and anticipation. Reduce tension by putting yourself to work. As the saying goes, "Don't count every hour in the day, make every hour in the day count."

WHAT DAD IS THINKING AND FEELING

Poet William MacNeile Dixon once wrote, "Birth is the sudden opening of a window, through which you look out upon a stupendous prospect. For what has happened? A miracle. You have exchanged nothing for the possibility of everything." What Dixon so eloquently captured is the essence of what it feels like to become a father. It is the feeling that you are ultimately unworthy to receive such a magnificent gift, yet desire nothing more than to get your hands on it. You are trying to savor your last days before the baby comes, while also looking ahead to the joy of finally being a parent.

It is common to feel the sudden urge to sprint or do 20 push-ups as excitement and energy periodically flood your brain. Such manic moments are natural after having waited so long to meet your child. On the other hand, it is also natural to, yet again, doubt your ability to be a good father or your willingness to revolutionize your lifestyle. You may also feel beside yourself with worry regarding your partner's health and ability to survive labor and delivery. These ups and downs are to be expected in the final weeks of pregnancy. However, the fear and doubt most men experience melt away within minutes of holding their newborn son or daughter. They are quickly consumed with what Dixon called "the possibility of everything."

THINGS DAD SHOULD KNOW

Your partner may experience pre-labor symptoms up to a month before actual labor begins. Pre-labor is a result of mom's cervix getting ready by dilating and effacing.

Pre-labor can often be confused with real labor, so it is important to know the difference:

Lightening: First-time moms may experience baby dropping into the pelvis from 2 to 4 weeks before labor begins. Women who have had previous pregnancies usually will not have this happen until real labor begins.

Abdominal cramping or pressure: Due to baby's presence in the pelvis, increased production of relaxin, and cervical dilation and effacement, mom may feel cramps similar in intensity to menstrual cramps. These are not contractions, however.

Static weight or weight loss: Mom will stop gaining weight and may even lose a pound or 2 as labor approaches.

Bleeding in these late weeks can be completely normal and is a result of minor injury to the cervix. This type of bleeding is usually light. It is pink or red and streaked through normal discharge. It generally occurs after intercourse or a vaginal exam and is not cause for concern. However, bright red spotting or heavy bleeding may be an issue with the placenta, which will require immediate medical intervention. And finally, any bleeding along with contractions may indicate labor has begun—so call your doctor.

Nesting: An old wives' tale suggests that the nesting instinct is evidence that labor is about to begin. But many women experience this urge to get ready for several weeks before the onset of labor—or not at all.

Increased vaginal discharge: Mom will see an increase in leukorrhea this month that may be tinged with mucus and/or blood as another indication that labor is on the horizon.

Bloody show: Blood and mucus sloughed off during cervical dilation and effacement may be present from 1 to 4 days before labor begins.

Mucus plug becomes dislodged: The mucus plug will come loose when mom's cervix is dilated and effaced enough to dislodge it. This may happen a few weeks before labor begins, or it may signify that labor has started.

Diarrhea and nausea: Within a few days of the onset of labor, many women have bouts of diarrhea and nausea or vomiting.

🔍 DID YOU KNOW?

Lunar Month 10 is different from the other lunar months in that it usually only deals with the first 2 weeks of the month. These are an exciting 2 weeks, however, because so much happens, including the birth of your baby! It is important to note that only 5 percent of babies are actually born on their due dates, so there is a possibility that your partner will still be pregnant even after you finish reading this book. It can help to remind yourself that you can see the light at the end of the tunnel—and that light is your sweet boy or girl!

Intensification of Braxton-Hicks contractions: These contractions, which mom has likely been feeling for some time now, will increase in frequency and intensity as she gets closer to starting real labor.

HELPFUL HINTS FOR DAD

As the weeks drag on, mom may be tempted to try and induce labor on her own. There are several methods touted on the Internet, but most are not recommended as they can cause undesirable side effects such as intense contractions, diarrhea, nausea, vomiting, and painful cramping without actually inducing real labor.

The most popular methods are reviewed below. Use them to counsel your partner if she feels compelled to try one of the following:

Nipple stimulation: If your partner had the contraction stress test, she knows that nipple stimulation can cause contractions by releasing the hormone oxytocin. Although several hours of nipple play per day could conceivably result in the onset of labor, it is not a recommended method. Overstimulating the nipples can cause intense, painful contractions.

Frequent sex and orgasm: As long as the doctor says it is safe, frequent sex is fine until mom loses her mucus plug or her water breaks. Do not have sex after this point, because the risk of exposing the baby to an infection is high. Check with the doctor about orgasm since it can stimulate contractions. The success rate of sex inducing labor is undocumented and anecdotal.

Walking: Your partner may want to walk for hours a day in hopes that it will put her into labor. As long as she has not been placed on activity restriction this is a fine way to pass the time. There is no evidence that walking causes labor to begin, but it is surely a good way for her to calm her nerves.

✖ TIPS & ADVICE

The biggest favor that you can do for yourself and mom at this point is to keep busy and let her rest. Stay busy by reading, watching movies, having friends over for chats, organizing the baby's room, or working on your pregnancy scrapbook. Keeping your minds off the Big Question: "When will mom go into labor?" will help you and your partner maintain your sanity. Nap, run mom a bath, and go to bed early. You both want to be well-rested and energized for the long haul of labor and delivery.

> ### ⓘ PREGNANCY FACT
>
> During delivery, contractions become less frequent, coming at 3- to 5-minute intervals and lasting for 60 to 90 seconds. Mom may feel a burning sensation as baby passes through the birth canal. It is not unusual for mom to fall sleep for a few minutes between contractions because of how exhausting labor is. Remember, your job is to offer encouragement and help keep her on-task. Pushing and delivery can last between 1 and 3 hours; it begins once the cervix is completely dilated and ends with the birth of your baby!

Castor oil: An old wives' tale suggests that taking castor oil will jump-start labor. However, there is no evidence to support this claim, and it can be harmful to mom and baby. Plus, it is easy to overdose, thinking that more increases chances of starting labor. Drinking more of it will only cause nausea, vomiting, diarrhea, and dehydration.

Teas and herbs: Raspberry leaf tea and certain herbs are thought to induce labor. However, since there are no studies to confirm the safety, it is best for mom to avoid herbal methods at this point. Remind her that she has come too far to do anything rash and risky!

Spicy foods: If mom can stomach spicy foods, she should certainly indulge now and then. But there is no evidence to support the old wives' tale that eating spicy foods induces labor. It probably does nothing more than increase heartburn.

Essential oils: It is never safe for a pregnant woman to ingest essential oils or get them anywhere near her vagina. Make sure she never puts essential oils in a bath. She can burn them in a diffuser if she insists on using them to any degree.

COMMON QUESTIONS THAT DADS HAVE

With just a few weeks left to go, it is likely that many of your questions have been answered by this point. Some, however, may be lingering:

What if the baby is overdue? Most doctors today will not let a pregnancy continue more than 2 weeks past the due date. If labor does not progress naturally, your partner will be induced. To induce labor, her cervic is first ripened. This can be done with drugs, creams, or by inserting a water-filled balloon into the uterus. Then, the amniotic sac will be artificially ruptured. The doctor may use a small, thin, plastic hook to make a tear in the bag of waters. Mom will feel warm fluid leak. Doing this may decrease the length of labor. Next, synthetic oxytocin will be administered intravenously. The drug Pitocin will be given to stimulate contractions. Because synthetic oxytocin can cause intense and frequent contractions, mom's labor will be closely monitored to make sure baby does not end up distressed from lack of oxygen.

Can our twins be born vaginally? Fifty percent of women in America carrying twins end up having a Cesarean delivery. However, that also means that half of all mothers birth their twins vaginally. It just depends on the size of the babies, where they are positioned, and mom's overall health.

HOW DAD CAN DEAL

Spend the time left before your baby comes starting a time capsule for him or her. This is a low-maintenance and satisfying way to

> ### ① PREGNANCY FACT
>
> If you are just dying for your doctor to make an educated guess about when mom will go into labor, ask him for your Bishop score. Your Bishop score is based on cervical dilation and effacement, which is given a score between 0 and 3; the station of your baby's presenting body part, which is scored from 0 to 3; and the level of softening and the position of the cervix, which is given a score from 0 to 2. If your Bishop score is 6 or higher, mom is likely to go into labor within the next week.

spend your days. Get a small chest or plastic storage container and fill it with items that best represent the time he was in the womb.

Items to include in a time capsule for your child include:

- Newspapers
- Political magazines
- Celebrity magazines
- CDs released the month your child is born
- Letters from you about how you feel about becoming a father
- Photos of your partner while pregnant
- Copies of movies you watched in the third trimester
- Books you have read during the pregnancy
- A popular toy or video game released this year
- Printouts of any ultrasounds
- Mom's pregnancy calendar
- A compilation of songs you put together to welcome your baby
- Before and after pictures of the nursery

When your child is old enough, he will appreciate the effort you put into memorializing the year he was born.

HOW DAD CAN HELP

The best way to help mom this month is to keep her relaxed through physical contact and pampering. Sex can be a component of your relaxation therapy, but do not make it the only goal. Spend time connecting with your partner in ways that may not necessarily lead to intercourse but that help her to release stress and tension.

Some examples include:

Give your partner a massage once a day until labor begins. These can be quick—10 to 15 minutes max. Switch areas of the body on different days, but her shoulders, feet, lower back, calves, hands, neck, and scalp will always appreciate a good rub.

Massage your partner's perineum, the skin between the vagina and rectum that stretches during delivery. This may be a little too intimate for some couples, but research indicates that women who massage their perineum are less at-risk for needing this area to be surgically cut during delivery (an episiotomy). You can turn this practical preparation into foreplay by taking over the job from mom until delivery.

Bathe your partner. If mom's mucus plug and bag of waters are still intact, she will benefit from daily warm baths. You can increase her enjoyment by bathing her with a wash cloth or loofah. Keep a cup bath-side to pour cascades of warm water down her belly and back.

Hug and kiss her often. Hugging and frequent kissing has been shown to elevate endorphins, the body's natural painkiller and mood elevator.

HOW DAD CAN BE INVOLVED

Review and practice the birthing technique you and your partner have decided to use. This includes setting aside time each evening to work on your partner's stages of breathing and discuss what props and tools she'll use to manage the pain of labor. Also, go over cues and signals, should verbal communication become impossible, and evaluate your partner's tolerance for various touch and relaxation techniques.

DAD'S RESPONSIBILITIES

Your main job this month is to stick close to home and stay in contact with your partner whenever you are away from the house.

"A truly rich man is one whose children run into his arms when his hands are empty."
~ Author Unknown

Labor & Delivery

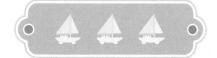

When you imagine your partner going into labor, it probably resembles the scene from the movie *Look Who's Talking*, when Kirstie Alley's character is rushed by taxi to the hospital. Her water breaks, and she hurls insults at John Travolta's character as he drives maniacally through traffic. When he tries to help her she violently snarls at him, "Stop touching me! I will have this baby without you touching me!" Indeed, your partner may become a little scary during labor. But you can reduce the overall stress for both of you by breaking labor and delivery down into smaller, more manageable steps. Doing so sets you up to know what to expect, how to prepare, and where to be flexible.

PACKING BAGS

Mom will probably want to pack her own bag, but since she might be forgetful and on edge at this point, it is a good idea to sniff around in her bag to make sure she hasn't forgotten any of the following:

- Non-skid socks and slippers
- Robe
- Nightgowns, which will be easier for her to labor in than pajama pants
- Nursing bras

Labor & Delivery . . . .

- Nursing pads
- Overnight-sized sanitary pads
- Several changes of underwear (pairs she won't mind getting blood stains on)
- An outfit to go home in
- Toiletries
- A pillow
- CD player and favorite CDs
- Portable DVD player and DVDs
- Magazines
- Labor tools (such as a tennis ball, aromatherapy oils, sock filled with rice, pillows, pictures of other kids or pets)

In your own bag, make sure to pack the following:

- Sweatpants or pajamas to sleep in
- Birth plan (up to 3 copies)
- Pillow and blanket
- Book, magazine, and newspaper
- Changes of clothes
- Camera and extra batteries
- Video camera
- Toiletries
- Cash
- Snacks, soda, or water
- List of people to call and their phone numbers
- Change to use a pay phone in case you do not get cell reception at the hospital
- Chargers for cell phones, CD, and DVD players

You can also put yourself in charge of packing a bag for your newborn. You'll want to include:

- Diapers
- Hats

- Booties or socks
- Mittens to prevent baby from scratching himself
- 5 or 6 receiving blankets
- Outfit to wear home
- Infant car seat

KNOWING TRUE FROM FALSE LABOR

Several of mom's symptoms will mimic true labor, so you'll want to be able to know when it's truly time to go and when you can still sit tight. Your partner will feel contractions in false labor, but these will be irregular. True labor involves regular contractions. The contractions in false labor do not intensify; in true labor, they become increasingly intense. Another difference between false and true labor contractions is that false labor contractions stay evenly spaced apart; true labor contractions get closer and closer together. Walking will relieve the discomfort from abdominal pain in false labor; walking won't do a thing for this pain in true labor. Finally, the cervix does not dilate in false labor the way it does in true labor.

WHEN TO GO TO THE HOSPITAL

When to go to the hospital is a question that must be decided by your partner's doctor, because the answer depends on your partner's health as well as the condition of the placenta when labor begins. Chances are your doctor has laid out a plan for when to go to the hospital. In normal, low-risk pregnancies mom is encouraged to do early labor at home. In this case, she will wait to go to the hospital until her contractions are 5 minutes apart for an hour, or after her water breaks.

Labor & Delivery . . . . 🦆

But if your partner is concerned that something is wrong, do not wait to get the OK from the doctor. Go to the hospital immediately and call on the way. It is always better to be safe than sorry once labor starts. The worst that can happen is mom will be sent back home if the hospital staff determines she is not ready to be admitted.

If you are still unsure when to go, call the doctor first with answers to these questions:

- Are the contractions getting more intense?
- Do the contractions come at regular intervals or follow a pattern?
- Are the contractions lasting longer with each wave?
- Are the contractions coming closer together?
- Has mom's water broken?
- How much fluid came out?
- What color was the fluid?
- What does the fluid smell like?
- How long ago did her water break?

There are times when you should get mom to the hospital first and ask questions later.

The following situations are considered emergencies and require immediate medical evaluation:

- Preterm labor that begins 3 or more weeks before mom's estimated due date
- Vaginal bleeding
- Severe abdominal pain
- Feeling less than 10 fetal movements in 2 hours
- Fever higher than 102 degrees
- Severe and sudden headache
- Seeing flashes of light or spots
- Sudden changes in vision

- Feeling weak or numb
- Difficulty speaking
- Pain when urinating
- Blood in urine
- Feeling the urge to pee but nothing comes out
- Any sense that something "just isn't right"

WHAT TO EXPECT UPON ARRIVAL

Getting to the hospital is probably going to be a frantic time for you. Everything that has happened over the past 266 or so days has been leading up to this moment. You have prepared for it, you knew it was coming, and still you feel overwhelmed with both panic and excitement. This is completely normal for dad, but do not expect this same level of frenetic energy to greet you at the hospital. The nurses and other hospital staff members see dozens of pregnant women in labor each week. They deal with nervous dads, crazy moms, and they take it all in stride. This may be maddening for you—but just try and remember that your once-in-a-lifetime experience is a daily (or more) occurrence for them.

Another thing you might not expect is that unless your partner's labor has progressed to an advanced stage, you will be required to stop in the admitting department before your partner is shown to a room. She will have to fill out forms and be admitted to the hospital before she can relax. This is true even if you pre-registered. It is frustrating, but it is also the way most hospitals operate, so prepare to patiently suffer through this part.

Next, mom will be taken to a room—which may or may not be where she will deliver the baby—so the staff can evaluate her contractions and measure the dilation and effacement of her cervix. She will change into a hospital gown and the nurse will ask her questions about when her contractions started and about her overall health and symptoms. The nurse will also check her blood pressure, pulse, temperature, and vaginal area for blood or leaking amniotic fluid. She will also listen to the baby's heartbeat and might hook mom up to a fetal monitor. Once all of this preliminary work is complete, the nurse will leave mom and dad alone to labor in private for awhile.

ARTICULATING THE BIRTH PLAN AND ACTING AS A GO-BETWEEN

Your partner will be so consumed by what is happening to her body she will likely be unable to pay attention to instructions or articulate her needs. Filling this gap as liaison between mom and the nurses—and later the doctor—is one of your most important jobs. Included in the go-between job description is the ability to articulate your partner's birth plan without alienating and insulting hospital staff.

You can make the staff aware of your birth plan by giving a copy of it to the nurse and asking for a few minutes to go over the plan with anyone who will be attending to the birth. You might also post the plan on the white board in your room. Commit important sections to memory so you remember mom's preferences when certain situations come up and let staff know you and your partner are flexible about altering the plan if needed. Avoid putting medical staff on the defensive by remaining civil when expressing mom's preferences. Request that all steps and procedures be explained to you and your partner before being carried out.

THE STAGES OF LABOR AND DAD'S ROLE

There are three stages of labor to contend with before you get to meet your baby. Understanding what they are, how they unfold, how long they last, what to expect from your partner, and what your role is during them will prepare you to best coach and support your partner.

Stage 1

The first stage of labor is broken down into three phases and is often the longest. It lasts between 12 and 16 hours. The three phases of Stage 1 labor include early labor, active labor, and transition.

Phase 1 is early labor which usually occurs at home. It lasts about 7 or 8 hours. During this time, the cervix dilates from 0 to 3 centimeters. Contractions are irregular, coming 5 to 15 minutes apart and lasting 25 to 45 seconds. For this reason, early labor is sometimes confused with false labor. But your partner will also experience aching back, abdominal cramping, and tightening of her uterus, which should make clear that this labor is true. Furthermore, she will have her bloody show, the mucousy bloody discharge that occurs when the mucus plug becomes dislodged. Her water may also break. During this period, you can expect your partner to be positive, talkative, and energetic.

During this period, encourage your partner to eat something. It may be a while before she can eat again. Urge her to stick to drinking water and make sure she conserves her energy. Taking a warm bath or shower can help relax her and, if it is possible, she should try and nap.

During this time, it is your job to write down when mom's contractions began and evaluate their progression. Time them, noting how long

Labor & Delivery . . . .

they last and how far apart they are. Let the doctor know that labor has begun. Until it is time to go to the hospital, you can keep your partner occupied by talking to her, playing a game with her, watching a movie, or by leaving her alone if she prefers. Use your time to make sure the hospital bags are in the car, the car has a full tank of gas, and that other children and pets are taken care of.

The second phase of Stage 1 is active labor. This phase is done partly at home and then completed at the hospital or birthing center. This phase lasts between 1 and 4 hours. During it, the cervix dilates from 3 to 7 centimeters. Contractions are 3 to 4 minutes apart and last 40 to 60 seconds each. Your partner can expect contractions to become progressively more painful for longer durations. At this point, mom may become nauseous and vomit, or she may have diarrhea. She may also feel very hot and sweaty.

At this point, she may hyperventilate or start to panic. It is likely that she will be extremely thirsty, but she can only have ice chips at this point. She will experience increased pressure and tightening of her uterus.

This is the time when your partner should bring in the breathing techniques she's learned. These will help her stay calm, focused, and help manage the pain. She'll need to let her body go with the contractions instead of fighting them—this will make pain worse. She should rest and conserve energy between contractions, and feel free to grunt and groan if it helps. This is the time to ask for pain relievers if she wants them.

For most dads, this is the point at which it gets increasingly difficult to witness labor, but you'll have to hang in there for mom's sake. Remind your laboring partner to focus on an external fixed object. Offer her the labor tools she's brought. Encourage her to walk, sit, take a shower, lie down—in other words, change positions as needed. Breathe with mom during contractions to remind her of the technique, and encourage her to switch techniques when they stop working. Keep suggestions and commands short as she is likely to have trouble processing them.

During this phase, be encouraging, but avoid cheerleading her. Being overly positive is likely to annoy her. Keep a cool cloth handy for her forehead and have some ice chips nearby. If she wants it, you can massage her or put pressure on her lower back to counter contraction pain. Above all, do not yell at her, cajole her, or freak out in front of her. Just stay calm and flexible, and give her plenty of space.

The third phase of Stage 1 labor is called the transition phase. This phase almost always happens at the hospital or birthing center unless a home birth was planned. It lasts between 30 minutes and 3 hours. During it, the cervix dilates from 8 to 10 centimeters and becomes 100 percent effaced. Contractions are very intense and may "double peak," coming every 1 to 2 minutes and lasting between 60 and 90 seconds each. Bloody show increases, and mom is likely to experience severe back pain and feel pressure on her bowels, rectum, lower back, abdomen, and vagina. She will have the urge to "bear down" and push and may hiccup, burp, pass gas, or even throw up. She may shake uncontrollably, be hot or cold, and may cry or scream.

She is also likely to become less cognizant of her surroundings and will have trouble following directions. Let her depend on you to guide her through this most painful stage of labor. You should offer continuous encouragement, and remind her that it is almost over! Give your partner 100 percent of your attention and get right in her face when giving her commands so she can really absorb what you are telling her. Remind her to breathe and stay calm. Make sure to communicate with the medical staff during this critical period so you can relay to mom any information or instructions.

Stage 2

Stage 2 of labor is the big show. It starts when mom is ready to push and ends with your baby's birth!

During this phase, pushing and delivery can last from just a few contractions to up to 3 hours. Contractions come every 3 to 5 minutes and last 60 to 90 seconds each. You can expect there to be more bloody show, and mom may feel a burning sensation as the baby moves through her pelvis. The urge to bear down and push intensifies and may cause mom to burp, pass gas, vomit, urinate, or defecate. Mom's perineum and rectum may ache, and she'll feel a stretching or possibly tearing sensation as baby moves through the birth canal. This may cause her to shake, spit, cry, yell, or grunt.

During this period, mom should follow all the doctor's instructions, pushing when told and riding out contractions. You should stay by her side and offer continuous encouragement. Help her count when pushing, as she will likely forget. Finally, after what feels like an eternity, the baby's head will crown, and shortly thereafter baby will be delivered from the birth canal. Your son or daughter will have entered the world!

Stage 3

Most people think labor ends with the birth of the baby—but it is not quite over yet. Stage 3 of labor includes delivery of the placenta. This stage lasts between 5 and 15 minutes. Contractions slow down and become less intense, and mom will be instructed to push as the doctor pulls to deliver the placenta. Her uterus will quickly shrink down to about the size of a grapefruit, and the doctor will check to make sure the placenta was delivered intact—any loose pieces could cause an infection inside of mom. Finally, your partner may be given a shot of Pitocin to keep contractions going long enough to shrink her uterus—unless otherwise specified in the birth plan.

During Stage 3, your partner should breathe, push, and listen to the doctor. Mom may be so ready to hold her baby or sleep, however, that she may not be interested in this phase at all. It certainly pales in comparison to what she just went through. Your job is to keep mom on task for just a little while longer. Tell her what a great job she did, and offer to hold the baby so she can rest. After you have all had a little bonding time, start making phone calls to announce the great news!

SHE DOESN'T MEAN IT!

Special mention must be made about mom's outbursts during labor and delivery. The woman you are with in labor may not even remotely resemble the woman you married. Birth is an ancient and animalistic process—it is no wonder that civility gets completely trampled when a woman is in the course of birthing a child. No matter how she yells, screams, or cries, treat her with respect, kindness, and patience.

Some women have reportedly told their husbands that they hate them, or wish they'd never been born. A woman who says such things under the duress of birth does not mean them—she is simply lashing out at an easy target. Just accept that during labor you may be insulted, cursed at, told to go away, pushed, punched, or growled at. Try not to take it seriously or personally, and remind yourself that your partner is in the greatest pain of her life—and that she loves you even though she hates you in the moment.

Labor & Delivery . . . .

PAIN-RELIEF MEDICATIONS

There is no denying that giving birth is painful—it is probably the most pain your partner will ever endure. However, studies show that resistance, fear, and lack of understanding significantly increase mom's pain during childbirth. Your job, therefore, is to help her understand labor so she doesn't try and fight it. You'll need to know what causes her to hurt and the different medications that are available for when it becomes too difficult to manage.

Pain during labor is caused by the many changes mom's body must go through to ready itself to push baby out. Some of the most painful changes are those that happen to the cervix—particularly during the transition phase when the cervix finishes dilating to 10 centimeters. Indeed, before your baby can be born, your partner's cervix must be thin and wide enough for her baby's head to fit through. For mom, this feels like sharp, stabbing pain in her vaginal area.

As this process unfolds over the course of several hours, painful uterine contractions cause lactic acid to build up, causing intense muscle pain and, in some cases, back labor. In addition, baby's head puts pressure on organs, bones, and joints as it passes through the birth canal. During delivery, all of these elements collide with the stretching and possible tearing of mom's vagina and perineum.

Your partner does not have to suffer, however. Thanks to advances in modern medicine, there are several pain relief options available to reduce or eliminate labor pain.

One class of such medications are called analgesics and narcotics. Of these, Demerol and Stadol are the most common drugs used.

They are given intravenously during the active phase of labor when the cervix dilates from 3 to 7 centimeters. These drugs help relax mom and reduce, but do not eliminate, pain. They tend to cause drowsiness, nausea, or vomiting, and may cause respiratory issues for baby when given close to delivery.

Another class of pain relievers are tranquilizers. Phenergan and Vistaril are the most commonly used drugs. They are given orally or intravenously during early or active phase of labor. They help decrease mom's anxiety and cause her to relax. They also eliminate the nausea caused by narcotics and improve narcotics' effectiveness. However, these drugs do not offer pain relief when used on their own.

The second most common type of pain reliever used is a sedative. Sedatives are given by mouth during early labor. Like the other medications, they relax mom and reduce her anxiety. They also stop false labor, cause drowsiness, but do not offer pain relief.

Local anesthetics might also be used. These are drugs that end in "caine," such as Lidocaine. Anesthetics are injected into mom's perineum to numb the area before an episiotomy when the baby's head is crowning. They only relieve pain at the site where it is injected and keep mom awake and able to push.

Another pain reliever is the Pudendal Block, which blocks the pudendal nerve from feeling pain. Lidocaine and Chloroprocaine are the most common drugs used to achieve this effect. They are injected into vaginal wall to numb the nerve and are given right before delivery of baby. The injection relieves pain in the vagina and rectum during delivery or for episiotomy while keeping mom awake so she is able to push. However, these drugs do not relieve pain caused by contractions. Furthermore, large doses may be required, and the drugs are ineffective on some women. Finally, they may inhibit baby's ability to breast-feed immediately after birth.

The epidural, or regional anesthesia, is probably the best known pain reliever. This is a combination of analgesics, narcotics, and medications to stabilize mom's blood pressure that are administered continuously through a catheter that is inserted into mom's spine. The epidural is given during the active phase of labor and may also be used for Cesarean deliveries. It blocks pain from the injection site to mom's toes but allows mom to be awake and alert. However, the epidural has several side effects to consider. For starters, your partner will be bed-bound, and it may be more difficult for her to know when to push. Epidurals also may increase or decrease the length of labor, decrease mom's blood pressure, or give her a "spinal headache." Also, there is a 15 percent chance it will only numb one side of mom's body.

Finally, there is the spinal block. This is when anesthetics or narcotics are injected once into mom's lower back. It blocks pain from the site and below and relieves pain for about 2 hours. It is mostly used for Cesarean births. It keeps mom alert and awake, but may lower her blood pressure, cause her to have trouble pushing, give her a severe headache, and the baby may have trouble breast-feeding immediately after being born.

Discuss with your healthcare provider the pros and cons of each type of pain reliever and the associated risks, and have an idea of your partner's preferences before you get to the hospital. These should be written in the birth plan you and partner came up with prior to heading for the hospital.

WHEN SOMETHING GOES WRONG

Even if mom's pregnancy has been low-risk and textbook, there is always a chance that something could go wrong during labor and delivery. Examples include failure of labor to progress, mom becoming unable to push without assistance, baby's head not fitting through mom's vagina, or fetal distress. In each of these cases, it is important not to panic, because your partner's doctor will be prepared to act swiftly by employing the following techniques or procedures.

Your doctor may try to facilitate labor if mom is having trouble. He may ask your partner to walk around the halls of the hospital, hoping that gravity will help the situation. Conversely, he may have mom rest and relax if she is too anxious for labor to progress. Labor-inducing drugs such as Pitocin (oxytocin), prostaglandin, and E-2 may be used to ready the cervix and stimulate labor progression. The doctor may also artificially rupture mom's amniotic sac.

The doctor may also use certain tools to help mom during the delivery. Forceps may be used if mom is having trouble pushing baby all the way out. Forceps look like large metal tongs and are inserted into the vagina. The doctor uses the forceps to gently grab hold of baby's head. The doctor gently pulls as mom pushes to help guide baby out through the birth canal. A vacuum extractor may also help during delivery. This device attaches to baby's head by a soft plastic cup. Suction is then used to gently pull baby out as mom pushes.

CESAREAN DELIVERY (C-SECTION)

More and more babies are being delivered by Cesarean section every year. A Cesarean, or C-section, is a surgical procedure in which the baby is taken out of the womb via an incision made by the doctor along mom's abdomen.

One-third of all C-sections are performed because labor has failed to progress naturally. Fetal distress, such as a drop in heart rate, low oxygen levels, or a twisted or compressed umbilical cord are other reasons why a C-section might be warranted. A C-section will also be performed if the baby is in breech position, or if mom has health problems such as preeclampsia, gestational diabetes, or vaginal herpes, which make it dangerous for her to give birth vaginally.

Being pregnant with multiples is yet another reason a doctor would perform a C-section, as are problems with the placenta, such as placental abruption or placenta previa. C-sections are also helpful in the case of umbilical cord prolapse, when part of the umbilical cord comes out before baby, cutting off his oxygen supply. Finally, if the baby is too large to fit through the birth canal, the doctor will delivery him by C-section.

Prior to undergoing the procedure, mom is prepped for surgery. She is given an antacid, and hooked up to an IV to receive medications and fluids. She will also be hooked up to machines that monitor her blood pressure and heart rate. A catheter will be inserted to drain her bladder, and her abdomen and vagina are shaved and made sterile. Then, an epidural or spinal block (or combination of both) is started.

Next she will be transferred to the operating room, where there may be up to 12 doctors and nurses present, including mom's doctor, an anesthesiologist, and a pediatric team. A screen is put up over mom's chest to block her view of the surgery. Dad will stand up near mom's shoulders after being outfitted with scrubs and mask.

When she is ready, an incision is made low in her abdomen. As the baby is lifted out of her uterus, she will feel tugging and pulling, but no pain. Once he is removed from her body, the baby's lungs are cleared and his respiration is checked. He is then presented to mom and dad, at which point dad may cut the umbilical cord. Finally, after the doctor delivers the placenta, mom is given an IV of antibiotics to prevent infection and is stitched up.

Recovery from a C-section occurs in several stages. In the first 24 hours following the procedure, your partner is moved to a recovery room where she will be monitored until anesthesia wears off— usually between 1 and 4 hours. She may breast-feed if she chooses, though many women sleep during the initial recovery period. As the epidural or spinal block wears off, your partner may feel cold, itchy, and have the shakes. She will be closely monitored by the hospital staff should any complications arise.

About 6 to 8 hours after the C-section, your partner will be encouraged to get up and walk around. She will be given pain relievers to manage the incision and afterbirth pains. She will be allowed to have food and drink about 24 hours after surgery. Mom can expect to recover in the hospital for 3 or 4 days following a C-section, and full recovery takes about 6 to 8 weeks. The stitches that were used to close up mom's internal incisions will self-dissolve, but external sutures or staples will likely be removed before she leaves the hospital.

Since a C-section qualifies as major abdominal surgery, remind your partner to rest afterwards. She can go on frequent but short walks but should, in general, be on activity restriction. She shouldn't lift anything heavier than the baby and should not drive for at least 2 weeks.

Finally, be prepared for some depression. Some moms feel "cheated" out of experiencing a vaginal delivery when they deliver via C-section. Assure your partner that she is every bit a mother as a woman who delivered vaginally. Indeed, the only thing she probably missed out on was excruciating pain. She might not see it this way at first, but her feelings of inadequacy will likely dissolve once she throws herself into caring for your newborn.

IMMEDIATELY AFTER THE BABY IS BORN

Whether your child is birthed vaginally or via C-section, the same basic sequence of events occurs immediately after he is born.

The following information will prepare you for what to expect in the minutes and hours after childbirth:

Cutting the cord: Soon after baby's delivery, you will have the opportunity to cut the umbilical cord. The doctor will clamp two sections of the cord and hold it up for you to cut—don't worry, he will talk you through it! Neither mom nor baby feels pain when the cord is cut. Do not feel pressured to do this if you don't feel up to it. The doctor will do it if you decide this experience is not for you.

APGAR test: One and five minutes after your baby is born, a nurse will assign her a score from 0 to 2 in each of the following categories:

- **Appearance:** The baby should be pink. If she is bluish or very pale, she will receive a 0. Mostly pink with some blue scores a 1, and pink all over earns a 2.

- **Pulse:** No heartbeat receives a 0. Less than 100 beats per minute gets a 1, and more than 100 beats per minute gets a 2.

• **Grimace:** If the baby does not respond to stimulation he receives a 0. If he shows mild irritation, a 1, and if he cries, a 2.

• **Activity:** Little to no movement receives a 0, some movement gets a 1, and constant motion gets a 2.

• **Respiration:** If baby is not breathing, his score is 0. If breathing is irregular or labored, he will be given a 1. Steady breathing and crying earns a 2.

Babies who receive a total score of 7 and above are considered healthy and thriving. Those who receive a score between 4 and 6 may need special care, including resuscitation and respiratory assistance. Babies who score below 4 will require serious medical intervention and may not survive. Most babies with an APGAR score below 7 will be transferred to the NICU for several weeks or months until they recover.

Holding baby for the first time: Holding your child for the first time can be emotional and a little scary. Don't be surprised if you are so overcome with emotion that you cry or shake. Don't worry that you will drop or break your baby—you won't. In fact, you will likely be surprised how natural it feels to have her in your arms.

Breast-feeding: Mom will likely want to start breast-feeding as soon as she is able. This is considered best for baby since he will be crying out for food and comfort. In addition, women who start nursing sooner rather than later tend to have greater success breast-feeding and bond with their child faster than those who wait. If this is your family's plan, let the nurses know that your son or daughter is not to receive any formula or be allowed to suck from a bottle. Also, request help from a lactation specialist to make sure mom has the maximum chance of success. Initially, your baby will feed on colostrum. This is a highly nutritious serum that satisfies your child until your partner's milk comes in. While mom is nursing, dad can observe, take pictures, rest, or get something to eat.

DAD TO THE RESCUE

Once word gets out that your baby has been born, your family and friends will want to flock to the hospital to take a peek. Well-wishers will be dying to bestow rubber duckies, balloons, flowers, stuffed bears, and other items upon mom and baby. Those who live too far to make the trek will be calling day and night to get updates on how mom and baby are doing.

This outpouring of care is overwhelming and will make you and your new little family feel special and loved. Some families will want everyone they know to come check out their new addition. Other families, however, feel uncomfortable being in the middle of a three-ring circus. Though your loved ones mean well, most people underestimate how exhausted dad, mom, and baby are in the hours and days after childbirth. This is why if you do not want people to swarm you after the birth, you should feel comfortable establishing the hospital as a "no visitors zone."

The best way to keep people away is to set aside 15 minutes or so to call a few key family members or friends. Say, "We're asking that people do not come to the hospital. Mom is trying to get the hang of nursing, and we're all exhausted. So, we would appreciate the time to rest, recover, and bond." Ask those you speak with to call others. Once the message is out, you will get what you need most: peace and quiet.

As for the people you do want to visit in the hospital—grandparents, aunts, uncles, and best friends, for example—ask them to call before coming over. This way, you can let them know if mom is sleeping or if the doctor is examining mom or baby. Let them know the best time to come by and ask them to limit their visit to about 15 minutes.

Taking on the role of "family bouncer" is not necessarily pleasant, but very important if privacy is what you want. Mom will probably be too polite to say, "Get out, I'm exhausted!" She'll be relying on you to intuit when lingering visitors need to be told to leave. You can also enlist the help of nurses who can stop people at the desk and call the room to announce visitors before allowing them to enter. Keep in mind, though, that nurses are busy doing their jobs and can't be counted on to be your receptionist. It's best if you step up and take charge of how much access to mom and baby you allow your loved ones while still in the hospital.

GOING HOME FROM THE HOSPITAL

Depending on your family's experience, leaving the hospital will either be a welcomed or feared change. If mom and baby have received great care from attentive and loving nurses, your partner may never want to go home! Indeed, for many new parents, the time in the hospital feels like a stay of execution before being cut loose to care for their baby on their own.

On the other hand, it can be common for parents to want to leave the hospital as soon as possible—especially if there are other children waiting at home. If your partner had an uncomplicated vaginal delivery, she and the baby may be released from the hospital as early as 24 hours after delivery. If your partner had a C-section, however, she will need at least 3 or 4 days in the hospital to recover before going home.

Labor & Delivery . . . .

Whether you are in the hospital for a few hours or a few days, the day you check out will be a busy one.

Since mom is still recovering from the birthing experience, you will be expected to take the reins on the following projects:

- Dress baby appropriately for the weather outside
- Pack up everyone's belongings
- Take whatever supplies the nurses offer, including diapers, hats, blankets, pacifiers, gauze pads, lotions, creams, etc.
- Have the car seat with you—otherwise the staff will not allow your baby to leave with you in your car
- Thank all the nurses and doctors who tended to your family

The First 24 Hours

Congratulations, dad! You have waited months for this very exciting day—the day you bring your baby home. As you step over the threshold with your baby for the first time, you are likely filled with the twin emotions that have plagued you for much of the pregnancy: excitement and terror. A third, powerful emotion is also likely to be present—an all-encompassing love you have never before felt so strongly.

The first day home with a newborn is very daunting if you are a first-time parent. Knowing what to expect will greatly boost your confidence. One of the first things to know about your baby is that she will go through 6 states of consciousness.

These different states of wakefulness and sleep have been fully documented by researchers, and knowing them will help you learn your baby's patterns and be better able to anticipate her needs:

Quiet alert: Baby is awake, but still. Her eyes may rest on a particular part of mom or dad's face, as if she is trying to memorize it. She seems content and is quiet, and she may coo a bit now and then. Your baby will spend about 10 percent of each day in this state during her first week of life.

The First 24 Hours . . . .

Active alert: Baby makes little cooing sounds and moves constantly. She looks all around the room and does not focus on any one thing. This state often indicates that your baby is getting fussy and may need to eat, be changed, or held. Paying attention to baby's cues while in this state may prevent prolonging the next state—crying.

Crying: All babies cry. Though everyone knows this, new parents are consistently surprised by how much their baby cries. The crying state indicates that your baby is trying to communicate a need. Go through the following list of questions to figure out what she is trying to say: Could she be hungry? Have I changed her diaper recently? Does she have a fever? Did a noise wake her up? Is she tired? Does she want to be held?

Drowsiness: Your baby will enter this state just before going to sleep and after waking up. She will move a little, but remain quiet. Her eyelids will be droopy and she will seem content. It is best to leave her be while in this state since she may still be tired and drift off to sleep.

Quiet sleep: In the first few weeks, babies spend up to 90 percent of their days asleep. Quiet sleep is one part of their normal sleep cycle. In it, a baby will be very peaceful, very still, and will rarely even move or twitch. Quiet sleep is often alarming for new parents because of how eerily still the baby is. If you are concerned, lean down to feel baby's breathing or put your hand lightly on her stomach to feel the rise and fall of her breath. As long as she is breathing, she is fine.

Active sleep: Every 30 minutes, your baby will alternate between quiet and active sleep. Active sleep is when baby drifts into the rapid eye movement (REM) state. You will see her eyes dart back and forth beneath her lids. Some babies even open and close their eyes while in this state. She might also fidget, smile, twitch, and make various other facial expressions and sounds. She may wake briefly and cry, but wait a while before you go to her, as she may drift back to sleep.

Many newborns sleep through their first few days of life only to wake up complaining they are hungry or to announce they are the proud owner of another dirty diaper. This can be alarming to new parents, who had no idea their baby would literally spend 90 percent of each 24-hour period asleep and the other 10 percent eating or pooping. Your baby's sleepiness can also make completing basic tasks—such as feeding—difficult, frustrating, and time-consuming. The best way to handle this is to adapt your schedule to hers, rather than the other way around.

WILL I BREAK MY BABY? HANDLING A NEWBORN

Picking up, holding, and carrying a 7-pound newborn can be terrifying. But following a few simple rules will turn you into a pro in no time. First, let your baby know you are about to pick him up. This way, you avoid startling him. When he is expecting your touch he is less likely to cry.

Once you've touched him a little, put one hand under his back and the other at the nape of his neck, cradling his head. Once you have your baby in your arms, cradle him in the nook of one arm, hold him against your shoulder, or use two hands to hold him against your abdomen. Your newborn will also like to sit against your chest while facing out toward the world around him. Try holding your baby in various positions to get used to them. It will also be fun to give him different perspectives on his environment. No matter what position you find he likes best, always remember to support his head and neck whenever you pick him up, for as long as you hold him. His neck is not yet strong enough to hold his head unsupported, and failing to support his head and neck can hurt him.

In addition to supporting his head and neck, always make sure you are aware of the two soft spots on his head, called fontanels. These are the areas where his skull has not yet closed. This area remains unfinished so baby's head can adjust while being squished through the birth canal and stays soft after the birth so his brain can grow. Though they are soft, the fontanels are not as vulnerable as you might think. Indeed, a thick, tough membrane stretches across each opening to protect your baby's brain from injury. The fontanel at the top of his head is approximately 2 inches wide and will begin to close at around 6 months of age. It does not completely close, though, until your child is about a year and half old. The other fontanel at the back of baby's head is less than half an inch wide. This one completely closes by the time baby is 3 months old.

When carrying your newborn, you can hold him in one of the above-mentioned ways or use a carrier that allows you to be "hands-free." Slings and front carriers are very popular because they allow parents to be mobile. Furthermore, the motion often lulls the baby to sleep. Many babies actually prefer to sleep in a sling because it is warm and snug and prevents them from moving their limbs involuntarily. Babies are also comforted by the sound of mom or dad's heartbeat and the rise and fall of their chest as they breathe. Therefore, wearing baby in a sling is an excellent way for you to bond with your newborn child. It also is a successful tool for soothing a fussy baby and allowing mom to get some rest.

BREAST-FEEDING

When it comes to feeding your baby, experts agree that the breast is the best. Breast milk is the perfect mix of fat, nutrients, and calories for a newborn baby. It is also easily digested and filled with important antibodies that help your baby fight infections. Other reasons you should encourage your partner to breast-feed include the fact that it releases hormones that helps mom's uterus shrink back down to its normal size, it burns up to 500 additional calories per day, and is a way for mom and baby to immediately bond.

While breast-feeding may seem like a job for mom and mom alone, there are several ways you can incorporate yourself into the ritual. Some new dads like to take on the job of bringing the baby to mom for feedings. While your child is nursing, you can sit close to mom, touch your baby's arms and legs, and take photos. You can also put yourself in charge of keeping a chart of feeding times and wet and poopy diapers. These help you and mom get to know your baby's habits. Finally, you can ask your partner to fill bottles of breast milk that you can feed to the baby while she is sleeping or out of the house.

Both you and your partner should expect that establishing a breast-feeding routine will take time, patience, and practice for mom and baby—and much encouragement from dad. A lot of moms are surprised to learn how difficult it actually is to get a handle on the right technique. You can keep your partner motivated by helping her research lactation methods, encouraging her to join a breast-feeding support group (where she might pick up some tips and tricks of the trade), and keeping her hydrated and well-fed to promote nutritious breast milk.

Should your partner choose to continue breast-feeding, she'll need to spend some time perfecting baby's position on the breast—called "latch"—and find the most comfortable position to nurse in. You

The First 24 Hours . . . .

can help her by having different nursing stations set up and ready to go. Examples include having a rocking chair or glider in the nursery, piles of pillows on the bed, and a comfortable chair with an ottoman near a television. Your partner will spend so much time nursing at first that she will probably want a few location options, a change of scenery, and some entertainment. Once her milk comes in, she can expect to be nursing her baby every 1 to 3 hours around the clock!

This means baby should not be allowed to sleep for more than 3 hours in a row between feedings, and not longer than 4 hours at night. There are two reasons for this—one is that baby requires this many feedings in a 24-hour period in order to gain weight, stay hydrated, ingest critical antibodies, and support her development. The second reason is that the only way for mom to build her milk is through supply and demand. Thus, the more often she feeds baby, the greater her milk supply. Plus, mom must empty her breasts every few hours so she does not develop a painful breast infection, such as mastitis. You can help mom and baby establish a feeding routine by bringing baby to mom for night feedings. Of course, you will all be so exhausted you may have to set your alarm for 4 hours after you go to bed to keep baby from missing a feeding.

It is especially important that mom not give up on breast-feeding during the first 24 hours home. During this time, the baby may not eat very much, but mom's milk will still be coming in. Encourage your partner to have patience during this initial period, because the benefits of breast-feeding are well worth it. Also be prepared for your baby to initially lose a bit of weight—up to 10 percent of her birth weight. This is normal, and she will regain it—and more—about 3 or 4 weeks after birth.

BURPING BABY

One way for you to participate in your baby's feedings is to burp her after she eats. With each feeding, your newborn will swallow a small amount of air that will cause her to feel gassy, bloated, and uncomfortable. It can be scary to smack the back of someone so small, which is why proper technique is important. Gently rub and pat your baby's back to help her pass air from her stomach. And don't forget to grab a burp cloth and lay it over your shoulder since you can expect to be doused with up to a tablespoon of spit-up at each burp session.

Several positions are effective for burping your baby. One is to sit her up in your lap. To get her in position, place your baby on your lap and lean her over your arm. Support her head by placing your hand under her chin. Rub or gently pat her back while continuously supporting her head.

You might also try laying your baby on your lap. Put her face down on your lap with her stomach over one of your legs and her head on the other. Gently rub or pat her back to get her to burp. Finally, you can try burping her against your shoulder. Hold her snugly against your upper half, and then gently pat or rub her back until she burps.

POOP AND MORE

In the first 24 hours after your baby is born, she will only produce enough urine to dirty a single diaper. As long as she is thriving and getting enough to eat, the number of dirty diapers will increase every day. For example, on the second day you can expect your baby to dirty two diapers; on the third, she will go through three of them. By the fourth day, she will require five or six changes a day.

The contents of your baby's dirty diapers will consist mostly of light-colored urine and dark, tar-like meconium for the first couple of days. But once mom's milk supply is stable, your baby's bowel movements will become yellow-mustard in color and have a seedy, runny texture. You can expect between three and four diapers per day to contain poop, while the rest are just wet. If you ever notice blood, diarrhea, or a maple syrup smell in your baby's diaper, call the pediatrician right away. A maple syrup smell can indicate a metabolic disorder that can be fatal. You should also call the doctor if baby does not produce at least five wet diapers a day after the fourth day of life.

FAMILY SLEEP

New parenthood means the addition of a baby equals the subtraction of sleep for mom and dad. Because your baby has to wake up so often to eat, her presence shreds any semblance of a normal sleep schedule. There are ways to minimize the impact on your family's sanity, though. While it will take a while for your infant to develop a sleep routine, you can inch your way toward that glorious day by figuring out what sleeping arrangements work best—and then be willing to change them when they stop working.

Your family's first priority is to get a handle on baby's feeding routine and then build a sleep schedule around it. By now you know that although your baby may sleep up to 16 hours a day, he also has to wake up to eat every 1 to 3 hours. And since it can take up to 45 minutes per feeding until mom and baby get the hang of nursing, there isn't much time left for rest. So whatever sleep you and mom do get must be quality rest. It is especially important for mom to get as much rest as possible while she recovers from childbirth.

Help you and your partner get quality rest by avoiding caffeinated beverages up to 8 hours before you plan to sleep. Skip the night cap—alcohol actually reduces the quality of sleep. If your baby is sleeping, you should be trying to sleep too—taking a few short naps is better than not sleeping at all. Furthermore, facilitate sleep by making the house a noise-free zone. Turn off the ringer on your home and cell phones, and invest in some good shades to keep light out so you can nap more easily. Turn off the TV, radio, and computer so you are not distracted, and put clean sheets and lots of pillows on your bed to make it an inviting place. Keeping the house temperature on the cool side will also help you sleep, as will exercising regularly.

Next you'll need to decide where your baby will sleep: in a bassinet near your bed, in a crib in her own room, or in bed with you and mom.

To make a choice, ask yourself (and your partner) the following questions:

- What are the pros and cons of each sleeping arrangement?
- When will each partner be going back to work (and needing to keep a more normal schedule)?
- How large a space do we live in?
- Do we mind having to go into another room for feedings?
- Are we comfortable with baby being alone in her own room?
- Can we sleep with the baby in a bassinet in our room?
- Does the baby seem content in the bassinet?
- Are night feedings easier with baby nearby or a little farther away?
- Will we bond better with baby if we co-sleep?
- Does the family bed arrangement make night

feedings quicker?

- Are we willing to try each option to see which works best, even if we lose sleep in the process?

It is important to note that the American Academy of Pediatrics (AAP) and the U.S. Consumer Product Safety Commission (CPSC) advise against allowing your newborn to sleep in bed with you. This arrangement risks a parent accidentally rolling over onto the baby or baby accidentally suffocating or being strangled by pillows, sheets, and blankets. Your baby could also fall or get accidentally pushed out of bed. Finally, research indicates there is a higher risk of Sudden Infant Death Syndrome (SIDS) in family bed arrangements. For all of these reasons, it is best to keep your bed for just you and your partner.

SWADDLING

Wrapping babies for sleep—or swaddling them—is an ancient practice that parents continue to use today. It restricts movement, keeps baby warm, and allows him to feel secure. Properly swaddling your baby for sleep is a bit of an art that you will perfect within the first week or two of bringing him home. It is an important art to master as it is the best way to keep your child from waking himself up by squirming around.

Swaddling is most effective during the first month when baby's movements are jerky. You will stop swaddling completely once your child is able to roll over, which occurs at around 2½ or 3 months old. While you'll want to swaddle often prior to that, leaving your baby swaddled for too many hours a day can inhibit muscle development and limit motor skills. Furthermore, swaddling when it is very hot out can increase the risk of SIDS.

To swaddle your baby, start with a thin, lightweight receiving blanket, preferably one that is square-shaped. Fold one corner down and place your baby in the center of the fold. Pull the left corner snugly across baby's chest, making sure that your baby's right arm is pressed against her side. Then, tuck the corner of the blanket under your baby's left side. Bring the bottom of the blanket up across her body to her chest, and hold her left arm against her side. Bring the right corner of the blanket snugly across your baby's chest and tightly tuck the blanket corner along her back. If you're having trouble with the process, search "how to swaddle baby" on www.youtube.com. There are many instructional videos posted there.

Swaddling will help your newborn sleep better, but it won't be enough to keep her asleep if you have a never-ending parade of visitors over to the house. It is important to set visitation restrictions so you, mom, and baby all get enough rest. Since you are all sleeping at different times of the day, it is best to ask all visitors to hold off on phone calls and visits until after the first week. However, if mom wants to see certain people during the first week, set a 45-minute time limit. Establishing this rule ahead of time will (hopefully) prevent visitors from lingering too long.

You can also keep drop-ins away by putting a sign on your door that reads, "Thank you for stopping by, but we are sleeping—please do not knock or ring the doorbell. Feel free to leave a note and we will call you when we are up to it. Thank you!" Leave a box of paper and some pens on the doorstep, and people are likely to respect your wishes.

WHEN THERE IS AN EMERGENCY

There is a chance that mom or baby may take a turn for the worst once home from the hospital. Knowing when to call the doctor and get to the emergency room is an important part of your role during the postpartum period. As the only one in the house who has not just undergone a major trauma, it is your responsibility to keep an eye on your partner and baby. Regularly ask your partner questions about how she feels and to share about her symptoms with you.

The following complications in your partner require a call to the doctor and/or a trip to the emergency room:

- Bleeding that persists longer than 4 days after childbirth
- Bright-red blood with large clots
- Feeling faint as a result of blood loss
- Signs of shock
- Fever
- Severe abdominal pain
- Greenish discharge from vagina, episiotomy, or C-section incision
- Redness, swelling, or increasing pain at C-section incision site
- C-section incision opens
- Unable to urinate
- Pain or burning sensation during urination
- Blood in urine
- Severe vomiting
- Severe headaches
- Shortness of breath
- Chest pain
- Coughing up blood

The following complications require a call to the doctor and/or a trip to the emergency room for baby:

- Will not eat
- Fewer than five wet diapers after the fourth day
- Blood in urine or stool

- Maple syrup smell in diaper
- Persistent vomiting
- Distended, hard belly
- Green discharge from umbilical cord stump
- Excessive crying or fussiness
- If dropped
- Respiratory problems
- If baby turns blue
- Fever
- All-over body rash
- Persistent diarrhea
- Lethargy
- Baby looks jaundiced or yellow
- Gut feeling that something is wrong

However, don't let yourself be consumed by fear of a trip back to the hospital. More likely is that your first 24 hours will be spent bonding and enjoying the wonder of being a family.

"Where there is love, there is life."
~ Gandhi

Notes . . . .

The First Month

There is a lot to figure during the first month after baby is born and, frankly, it can be overwhelming for a first-time dad. First, you have to learn how to take basic care of a tiny human being—including how to feed, burp, clothe, diaper, bathe, and handle him. Next, you try to make sense of your new role as a father and how it impacts your relationship with your partner, not to mention your sex life. Throughout this time, you battle fears of breaking or dropping your baby, losing him to SIDS, and going back to work. Finally, if you have other children or pets, you are likely stressing about how to keep them happy while you and your partner adjust to having a newborn. Compounding the issue is the fact that all of these issues are yours to process on very little sleep—which makes these first few weeks very challenging.

Yet the first few weeks home with your baby and partner are also among the most magical you will ever experience. You have bonded with your partner in an unprecedented way. Watching her labor and birth your child solidified the deep bond you feel with her, and it is likely you love her more than you ever have. That love is physically represented in the child you have created together, whom you look at dozens of times a day and think, "How did I get so lucky?!"

The First Month . . . . 🦆

YOUR PARTNER'S RECOVERY

If your partner isn't on the same page as you, it is because her body is still reeling from the after-effects of childbirth. Over the next several weeks, you can expect her body to go through many stages as it works to return to its pre-pregnancy state. How quickly mom heals depends on her birth experience and how much support she gets from you as she recovers.

Over the course of the next 6 weeks—called the postpartum period—mom will go through the following changes:

Afterbirth pains: In the first 3 to 5 days after mom gives birth, she will experience afterbirth pains. These are uterine contractions that shrink her uterus back to its pre-pregnancy size. They feel like menstrual cramps and won't be nearly as intense as the contractions she endured during labor. Breast-feeding releases the hormone oxytocin, which causes the contractions.

Uterus changes: When she went into labor, your partner's uterus weighed between 2 and 2½ pounds. Over the next 6 weeks, it will shrink back to its pre-pregnancy weight of about 2 ounces. As long as mom breast-feeds, she will not resume menstruating until about 12 weeks after childbirth, though some women get their period as early as 7 weeks after. Still, other women find their menstrual cycle is delayed for as long as they nurse—up to a year.

Vaginal changes: Your partner's vagina, stretched by childbirth, may be sore for 6 to 8 weeks after delivery—especially if she had an episiotomy. If so, it may take up to 3 months for her to heal. This makes sitting uncomfortable and sex out of the question. In addition, mom's vaginal muscles are stretched out and weak. To tighten them, she should perform Kegel exercises when she feels up to it. She will also experience vaginal dryness as long as she breast-feeds, since nursing decreases the amount of estrogen her body produces. However, mom will experience significant vaginal discharge called lochia for about 4 weeks. During the first 4 days, lochia is similar to menstrual blood. Then it changes to a thicker, yellowish fluid.

Breast changes: Mom's breasts will leak and be sore for as long as she is breast-feeding, but particularly when her milk first comes in. This can happen in a rush, filling her milk ducts and causing hard, tender lumps. The best cure is for her to continuously nurse to move the milk through and clear the ducts. If, however, your partner's breasts become red and hot to the touch, she has probably developed mastitis—a painful infection that may require medical attention. In addition, mom's nipples may become dry and cracked and may even bleed. She should treat them with her own breast milk or with special ointment for breast-feeding moms.

Your partner's body will change in a few other ways as it searches out its pre-pregnancy self. It is embarrassing, but mom may leak urine for a few weeks after delivery until her bladder recovers from the trauma. She also may be constipated for 2 to 4 days after giving birth and may want to take a gentle stool softener. In general, her entire body will be sore from giving birth, causing her to feel achy and weak. Her skin may get blotchy or broken out as her hormones readjust, which may also cause her to suffer bouts of night sweats. Finally, she can expect to lose up to 25 pounds of fluid immediately, as well as a significant amount of hair in the weeks after childbirth.

If your partner had a Cesarean section, you can expect her recovery to take about 8 weeks. As mom's body heals, she will experience several uncomfortable side effects in addition to most of the aforementioned body changes. For these reasons, it is especially important that you be willing to take on most—if not all—household chores to allow your partner to rest and heal.

Over the next several weeks, you can expect your partner to experience the following symptoms:
Painful gas and bloating for the first 36 to 48 hours after delivery. This can be reduced by taking frequent walks, avoiding gassy foods or carbonated beverages, and passing gas instead of holding it in.

Pain at the site of the incision for several weeks. This pain is excruciating at first, but lessens over time. Mom should take pain medication and rest when possible. She should not lift anything heavier than the baby. She should not do activities that engage the abdominal or lower back muscles. She should not exercise until at least 8 weeks after surgery (walks are OK). Also, mom should brace herself against a wall or hold a pillow to her abdomen when sneezing or coughing.

Itching at incision site for several weeks as it heals. Mom should keep her incision clean and dry and avoid scratching it.

BASIC CARE OF A NEWBORN

Newborns are actually very easy to take care of—it is when babies become highly mobile children with opinions that life gets really difficult. So, try and look upon the first few weeks of your child's life as a stroll down Easy Street. Someday you will laugh about how nervous you were—but to get to that point, of course, you need to know a few basic caregiving techniques.

Bathing

It is not necessary to bathe your newborn more than once every 2 or 3 days since he spends most of his time asleep. After that, don't submerge your baby in water until the umbilical cord stump is completely healed. A sponge bath will keep your baby clean and the umbilical cord stump site healthy. Most newborns do not enjoy having a sponge bath because they get cold easily and would rather be eating or sleeping.

You can reduce your newborn's discomfort by following these simple steps:

- Have all bath materials ready before getting your baby
- Make sure the water is warm, not hot
- Wash your baby in an infant bathtub, on the changing table, or on a waterproof pad on the floor
- Have access to both soapy water for washing and plain water for rinsing
- Have a soft wash cloth on hand, several sterile cotton balls to clean her eyes, no-tear baby soap, a hooded towel, as well as a clean diaper and pajamas
- Dip washcloth in warm, soapy water and clean baby's feet
- Work your way up or down his body
- Avoid wetting the umbilical cord stump
- If the room is not heated, expose only the area you are cleaning, and then rinse, dry, and cover him back up so he does not get cold
- If the room is warm enough for baby to be nude, wrap him in a hooded towel after his bath
- Expect your baby to pee (especially boys) when his diaper is off
- Only wash your baby's hair with baby shampoo once a week to avoid drying out his scalp

The First Month . . . . 🦆

Dressing

Putting clothes and pajamas on a newborn is simple. Just be gentle, and never try to force anything over your baby's head. Always dress your child on a stable surface, such as your bed or on a changing table. Never leave him unattended, either—not even for a moment. All it takes is a second for him to roll off the bed or table. Choose clothing with easy-access snaps for quick diaper changes. Note that most baby clothes correspond to a baby's age and are usually sold in ranges, such as "newborn to 3 months." Given this, your child may be slightly smaller or larger than his corresponding clothing.

Trimming baby's nails: For anyone who has accidentally cut the quick and made their dog bleed while trimming their toes up, the idea of cutting a flailing newborn's teeny tiny nails may be completely terrifying. However, you'll be surprised by how soft your baby's nails are. In fact, you won't have to use clippers during the first 6 weeks of life. Instead, you can simply peel the tips of the nails away when they become too long. His nails will grow fast, so you'll have to trim them every week or so. Peeling them away does not hurt, and you will not cause any bleeding. Trimming baby's nails is a must, because if they get too long, he will use them to scratch his face and eyes.

If you are too nervous to clip or peel his nails, enlist the help of your partner and make it a two-person job. If neither of you can stand to do it, keep your newborn's hands covered with little mittens for part of the day. This will protect him from accidentally clawing himself. This is not a permanent solution, of course, so at some point one of you will have to trim his nails. If you do nick baby's finger, do not use a Band-Aid: Your baby could choke on it. Instead, put pressure on the cut with a sterile cotton ball until the bleeding stops.

Doctors appointments: Your pediatrician will want to see your infant between one and three times in the first 6 weeks of her life—maybe more often if mom and baby are having trouble with breast-feeding or if there are health issues. Assuming everything is progressing normally, your baby will have at least one, but most likely two well-child checkups. In addition to making sure baby has regained his birth weight by the third week after being born, the doctor will also ask about baby's feeding, sleeping, and potty habits. Questions will be asked regarding his overall demeanor and movements. His weight, head circumference, and length will be measured, and his vision and hearing will be checked. The doctor will look at the umbilical cord stump site to make sure it is healing properly. If a Hepatitis B vaccination was not given at the hospital, your doctor will give it now. Finally, your pediatrician will have the results of any blood tests that were performed on baby in the hospital, such as a PKU screening, which checks for metabolic disorders. Finally, a circumcision may be performed if you have requested one.

Circumcision care: Originally developed as a religious rite of passage, circumcision is now a common procedure performed on male babies in the United States. Caring for a freshly circumcised penis is as easy as caring for the umbilical cord stump. It is important to keep the penis clean and dry, but you also must prevent it from sticking to his diaper. To prevent sticking, swab some Vaseline on the part of the diaper that will touch baby's penis. It is likely he will have gauze on the wound for several days until it falls off. He will be sore for a few days, but frequent nursing will help keep his mind off the pain. Your baby may ooze a yellowish fluid or even bleed a little until the penis heals, but it is nothing to be alarmed about. However, should he still seem to be in a lot of pain by the third day, or the site is oozing green or foul-smelling fluid, he probably has an infection and must see the pediatrician for treatment.

Umbilical cord stump care: When the umbilical cord was cut, your baby was left with a nub that probably looked a like a short blue-and-white tentacle sticking out of her belly. Over the course of the next 3 weeks, this stump will shrink, blacken, become crusty, and eventually fall off on its own. There is little you need to do to care for it other than keep it clean and dry. Do this by sticking to sponge baths and allowing the site plenty of air exposure. There is no need to apply alcohol to the area as it heals. Just leave it alone and let nature do its job. If the stump irritates your baby, you can fold her diaper down below her belly button.

Pay attention for signs of infection, and if any of the following symptoms develop, call the pediatrician:

- Stump is red and swollen
- Area around the site is swollen and red or hard
- Site persistently bleeds
- Green or yellow discharge
- Foul-smelling discharge

WHAT TO EXPECT FROM YOUR PARTNER

Your partner just went through a significant physical and emotional ordeal that consisted of 10 months of pregnancy and ended with the Herculean effort of giving birth. For the next 6 weeks you should understand that she will be tired and sore as her body readjusts to its pre-pregnancy condition. You can also expect her to have some emotional healing to do as well. She will probably cycle through many moods, including periods of depression. She may feel close and intimate with you, even needy, or be physically distant and focused solely on the baby. Your job during this time is to pay attention to her symptoms and how long they last. This will help you determine if your partner is suffering from baby blues, postpartum depression, or postpartum psychosis.

The Baby Blues: It is normal for mom to experience a "crash" during the first week after baby is born. After all, she is exhausted, recovering from childbirth, and her hormones are still all over the place—not to mention that she is trying to get the hang of breast-feeding and caring for a newborn. After all she has been through, she may not feel up to the challenge. In fact, 60 to 80 percent of new mothers experience these feelings, collectively known as the "baby blues." Other symptoms of the baby blues include insomnia, undereating, overeating, excessive worrying about baby, irritation and weepiness, sadness, and despair. In short, mom is bummed.

You can help mom get through the baby blues by cheerleading her efforts to breast-feed or supporting her decision to stop. Many parents are surprised to learn that breast-feeding does not come naturally to every mother or to every baby. In most cases, there are hurdles to jump over before nursing becomes stable and routine. It is common for women, especially those who had Cesarean deliveries, to experience delayed or low milk supply. Some women also have flat, inverted, cracked, or bleeding nipples, which makes it too painful to nurse. They might not be able to get their baby to latch properly to their breast. Mom might also develop thrush, a painful yeast infection in her nipples. Should the combination of these challenges make it too difficult for mom to breast-feed, she might feel like a failure.

Difficulties with breast-feeding can be demoralizing and will cause the baby blues to linger beyond what is normal. Also, societal pressures to keep at it may increase mom's level of guilt and cause her to become angry with herself. This, in turn, exacerbates the blues and may even turn into full-blown postpartum depression.

If your partner has difficulty breast-feeding, monitor her level of sadness, guilt, and frustration over the next several weeks. She should be in a better mood within 2 weeks after giving birth. If not, she may have crossed over to postpartum depression, and you'll want to be aware of it.

Postpartum Depression (PPD): Postpartum depression is a serious condition that affects between 10 and 20 percent of mothers. It lasts much longer than the baby blues—from several weeks to up to a year after childbirth. Because PPD usually sets in a month or two after baby is born, it is entirely possible that your partner will have the baby blues for a couple weeks, feel better for awhile, and then develop postpartum depression.

The likelihood of this occurring increases if she meets the following criteria:

- Experienced depression before becoming pregnant
- Was depressed during pregnancy
- Has a history of mental illness
- Developed PPD after a previous birth
- Has a family history of PPD
- Suffered from severe PMS
- Had a difficult pregnancy with or without bed rest
- Had an emergency Cesarean delivery
- Had a difficult labor and vaginal delivery that did not go as planned
- Has limited mobility while recovering
- Has had difficulty breast-feeding
- Has a baby who developed health problems
- Has a baby who was born with unexpected birth defects
- Has severe financial concerns
- Has a history of abuse
- Has relationship problems or is recently divorced

Postpartum symptoms include:

- Irritability
- Insomnia
- Panic attacks
- Anxiety
- Fear
- Excessive sleeping
- Increased or decreased appetite
- Frequent crying spells
- Feeling sad all the time
- Unable to take care of self or baby
- Disinterest in baby and other children
- Memory problems
- Excessive worry for baby's well-being
- Not showering or dressing
- Refusing visitors

Though some of the symptoms of PPD and baby blues are similar, PPD is much more serious and lasts a lot longer. This is why it important that you note whether mom's symptoms extend beyond 2 or 3 weeks. If they do, she needs treatment. The good news is that PPD is treatable with medication, therapy, or both. The key to managing PPD before it damages mom's relationship with baby and dad, however, is timely professional intervention.

Postpartum Psychosis: Postpartum psychosis is a rare condition that develops suddenly within the first 3 months after childbirth. It is a dangerous condition that, if left untreated, has a 5 percent suicide rate and a 4 percent infanticide rate.

Symptoms generally appear out of nowhere after a brief optimistic period and include:

- Hallucinations
- Suicidal thoughts
- Thoughts of killing baby
- Mania
- Delusions
- Panic attacks
- Severe anxiety
- Insomnia
- Illogical ideas
- Refusing meals

Women who have suffered from postpartum psychosis before are up to 50 percent more likely to develop this condition with subsequent pregnancies. Moms are also at a heightened risk if they suffer from psychosis, schizophrenia, or bipolar disorder. A family history of psychosis, schizophrenia, or bipolar disorder also increases a woman's risk of developing postpartum psychosis, as do severe feelings of isolation, severe financial problems, a recent tumultuous move or job change, and extremely low self-esteem.

Postpartum psychosis is a medical emergency that requires immediate hospitalization to prevent mom from harming herself or baby. It is treated with antipsychotic drugs and other medications and requires close supervision by an experienced professional.

Sex with a Recovering Partner: After the birth of his child, a man's sex drive may take several turns. After witnessing such a dramatic event as childbirth, some men are intimidated to be physically involved with their partners. Some feel guilty about having "caused" the process their partner has just endured, while others are a bit grossed out. Still others realize that their partner is now a mother, which reminds them of their own mother, which turns them off to sex.

Other men are eager to resume a normal sex life. It's been months since they've been able to be intimate with their partner in the way they want, and they are very ready to get back in the saddle. But even if you are ready to have sex again, your partner may not be. When (and whether) your partner is ready depends on several factors, including how long it takes her body to recover, her emotional state, her fear of becoming pregnant again, and whether she feels supported by you in the postpartum period.

Doctors generally recommend that women wait at least 6 weeks before resuming intercourse to allow their bodies time to heal. Yet many women don't see their sex drive return for many weeks after that, or even for a year until after the baby is born. One major reason your partner may not be interested in sex is that the birth and postpartum period have left her feeling completely asexual. She is exhausted, unhappy with her appearance, and feels claustrophobic from being pawed by a newborn all day long. In addition, your partner's breasts may be sore and leak, and feel much more functional rather than sexual. Finally, breast-feeding mothers will experience vaginal dryness as well as thinning of vaginal walls due to decreased estrogen production. None of these conditions are ripe for feeling sexual.

These physical reasons, plus the emotional rollercoaster that accompanies hormonal readjustments, may delay a normal sex life for longer than you expected. This can be frustrating for dads who thought sex would be in plenty soon after pregnancy was over. Pushing the issue is more likely to alienate your partner than encourage intimacy. Be patient and supportive with her—and know that sex will once again become a regular feature of your relationship once she makes a full recovery.

FEAR OF SIDS

There are few scenarios that strike fear deeper into the hearts of new parents than the possibility of losing a baby to Sudden Infant Death Syndrome (SIDS). In truth, SIDS is the leading cause of death in babies less than 12 months old. Over the years, SIDS researchers have been unable to predict whether a particular child is at-risk; however, they have identified certain factors that seem to increase or decrease incidences of SIDS. For example, mothers who smoke while pregnant are three times more likely to lose a baby to SIDS. Exposure to secondhand smoke also significantly increases baby's risk of succumbing to SIDS. You and your partner should take steps to make sure your baby is as safe as possible by following the guidelines suggested by the First Candle SIDS Alliance.

The "Back to Sleep" campaign that began in 1994 has reduced SIDS incidences by 50 percent each year. This campaign recommends always putting your baby to sleep on his back and checking him frequently to make sure he stays that way. Side- and tummy-sleeping babies are at high risk for SIDS. Make sure the mattress on which he sleeps is firm, and remove all stuffed animals, pillows, blankets, and loose sheets from his crib. Fitted sheets should snugly cover the mattress and should not come loose. Bumpers should not be used since they increase risk and are unnecessary for your child at this point. Never allow baby to sleep on waterbeds or couches, and never leave a hat on your child while he is sleeping, as it may cause him to overheat. Keep baby from overheating in general by keeping his room cool and dressing him appropriate to the current temperature. Also, always put your baby to bed with a pacifier. Pacifiers seem to significantly reduce the risk of SIDS because they prevent baby from falling too deeply into sleep. Pacifiers may also prevent him from rolling over onto his stomach.

The family bed sleep arrangement is considered unsafe by SIDS experts. Babies are at risk for suffocating or being strangled by blankets, pillows, sheets, and mom or dad rolling over on him. On the other hand, having baby sleep in a bassinet or crib in the same room as mom and dad may reduce the risk of SIDS, though researchers are not sure why. Finally, babies who are breast-fed for at least the first 6 months of life are at a significantly lower risk for SIDS. Keep these things in mind as you go about the first few weeks and months with your newborn.

GOING BACK TO WORK

Most men return to work within the first 1 to 3 weeks after baby is born. You may find this either a welcome return to normalcy or a difficult transition. Either way, there are some practical tips for making this change easier for you and your partner.

Ease back in to a full-time schedule. Before diving back into a 40-hour workweek, ask your boss if you can telecommute part of the week. Ask to spend 20 hours a week in the office and 20 working from home. Once back at work, stick to a regular schedule. For the first several months, avoid taking business trips and working late. This is a critical time to bond with your baby. Besides, mom will depend on you to relieve her.

Also, arrange for your partner to have help. Call on grandmothers, other relatives, and friends to spend a few hours with mom every day so that she can shower, rest, and eat. Getting time to herself every day will greatly reduce mom's stress level and make her less prone to depression once you return to work. And finally, check in often. Though you are not home, you can still feel like you are there by calling, emailing, or even texting home several times a day. It will make you feel good and keep you connected and updated on baby's progress. Ask her to email pictures of baby or to give you a couple updates over the course of the day.

"My life has been the awaiting of you.
Your footfall was my own heart's beat."
~ Paul Valery

Conclusion

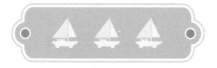

A Final Word

You may feel surprised by how different you actually feel now that your long-awaited child has been born. During the pregnancy, you sensed that major changes were brewing, but you could not have foreseen that your lifestyle—as well as your entire perspective—would shift so completely. Sure, you sensed the seriousness of the responsibility that was coming—you just didn't know what it would actually look and feel like until now.

As you adjust to the perils, joys, annoyances, and hilarity of fatherhood, remember that being a father is a process and a role that unfolds over the course of your entire life. Don't expect it to all come to you in one revelation. Let yourself off the hook to experience parenthood as it happens. Therefore, focus on adapting to keep up with your baby's constant changes.

Also, remind yourself that if you can't relate to your baby in the stage he is currently in, he will soon hit another phase of life for which you will be just the thing he needs. This is an important bit of advice for new dads to take to heart, as the first few months, even year, of baby's life he is intrinsically linked to mom. Baby relies on mom to feed him, and it is from this activity that much of their bond flows. Furthermore, it is most often the mom that stays home with baby, giving them more hours to bond a day than you.

Conclusion . . . .

But as your baby is weaned, you will come to have a special role in his life, one that no one else can fill. Remember that, as your baby grows, he is constantly watching you and looking up to you. You love him and set an example for him as only a father can.

Over the course of your partner's pregnancy, you probably heard the phrase, "Having a baby changes everything," at least 100 times. But now that you are actually living it, the biggest changes have become reality. One of the biggest changes new dads have a hard time adjusting to is the switch from a couple to a unit. The welfare of this unit must always be put before your own desires. It should not take too long for this new reality to settle in, as you have been grooming for this transition since the day your partner announced she was pregnant. Even so, life feels different, because it is. Whether you have become a three-, four-, or even five-person household, your role as a man has definitely evolved into something more than before your baby's arrival.

Figuring out just what this "something more" entails will take time. One thing for sure is that you have just added to your plate the tremendous responsibility to provide for—and take care of—your entire family unit. This responsibility can be overwhelming and joyous all at once. Sometimes you will feel in over your head and even sure you are destined to fail.

But, in actuality, you have been preparing for this change your entire life. In fact, learning to be a father began with first being a son. As a son you learned what a child needs from his father and watched as your dad figured out how to meet those needs. You learned to integrate his successes and how not to repeat his failures. Since you are used to looking at fatherhood from the perspective of a child you may feel like an adolescent pretending to be a grown-up. Feeling like a parental impostor is very common and, if you discuss it with your partner, it is likely she feels the same way.

Try to avoid falling into the new dad trap—the one in which you feel like an amateur who always defers to mom as the expert since she handles the majority of baby's basic care. In truth, mom is learning as she goes, as you are. By talking it out together you realize how connected to each other you are by the unfamiliar experiences of new parenthood. Roll up your sleeves and do not be afraid to get your hands dirty. Jump in and feed, diaper, dress, bathe, hold, and play with your child. Make an effort to read to him and put him down for naps and bedtime. Doing all of these things with your child daily establishes your role of involvement from birth, vastly improves your self-confidence, and chisels away lingering feelings of inadequacy. What surfaces in its place is your commitment to rise up, accept the added responsibility, and strive toward greatness— as a father, a partner, and a man. For as Sir Winston Churchill once said, "The price of greatness is responsibility." Since there is no more important responsibility for a man than fatherhood, you are most certainly destined for greatness.

"Any man can be a father.
It takes someone special to be a dad."
~ Author Unknown

Notes . . . .